About the Author

Barbara Aehlert is the President of Southwest EMS Education, Inc. in Phoenix, Arizona and Pursley, Texas. She has been a registered nurse for more than 30 years with clinical experience in medical/surgical and critical care nursing and, for the past 21 years, in prehospital education. Barbara is an active CPR, First Aid, ACLS, and PALS instructor. She is the Director of Field Training for Southwest Ambulance in Mesa, Arizona, and an active member of the Pursley, Texas, Volunteer Fire Department.

Index of Topics

A

E

F

G

Introduction to Emergency Medical Care

The Emergency Medical Services System

- A healthcare system is a network of people, facilities, and equipment designed to provide for the general medical needs of the population.
- The Emergency Medical Services (EMS) system is part of the healthcare system. It consists of a coordinated network of resources that provides emergency care and transportation to victims of sudden illness and injury.

Levels of Prehospital Education

- There are 4 levels of nationally recognized prehospital professionals: Emergency Medical Responder (EMR), Emergency Medical Technician (EMT), Advanced EMT (AEMT), and Paramedic.
- Emergency Medical Responders and EMTs provide Basic Life Support (BLS). Advanced EMTs and Paramedics provide Advanced Life Support (ALS).

Medical Oversight

- Every EMS system must have a medical director. A medical director is a physician who provides medical oversight and is responsible for making sure that the emergency care provided to ill or injured patients is medically appropriate.

- On-line medical direction is direct communication with a physician by radio or telephone, or face-to-face communication at the scene before a skill is performed or care is given.
- Off-line medical direction is the medical supervision of EMS personnel by means of policies, treatment protocols, standing orders, education, and quality management review.

Quality Management

- Quality management is a system of internal and external reviews and audits of all aspects of an EMS system.
- Quality management is used to identify areas of the EMS system needing improvement. Quality management helps to make sure that the patient receives the highest quality medical care.

Phases of a Typical EMS Response

The phases of a typical EMS response include:

- Detection of the emergency
- Reporting the emergency (the call made for assistance, dispatch)
- Dispatch/response (medical resources sent to the scene)
- On-scene care
- Care during transport
- Transfer to definitive care

Types of Specialty Centers

Burn Centers

Burn centers specialize in the care of burns ranging from relatively mild to life-threatening burn injuries. Services include helping the patient and family with the emotional stress that often comes with a burn injury and daily assistance with exercise, scar control, wound care, splinting, and activities of daily living.

Heart/Cardiovascular Centers

Heart and cardiovascular centers specialize in treating disorders of the heart and blood vessels.

Hyperbaric Centers

Hyperbaric centers specialize in hyperbaric oxygen (HBO) therapy, which uses the administration of 100% oxygen at a controlled pressure (greater than sea level) for a set amount of time. Carbon monoxide poisoning and smoke inhalation are 2 conditions that may be treated with HBO therapy.

Pediatric Centers

Pediatric centers have trained professionals that recognize the medical, developmental, and emotional needs of children. Children are not just small adults. Their bodies are different, and the illnesses and injuries they experience often produce signs and symptoms that differ from those of an adult.

Perinatal Centers

Perinatal centers specialize in the care of high-risk pregnancies.

Poison Control Centers

Poison centers specialize in providing information in the treatment of poisonings and drug interactions. Some poison centers also provide education programs for medical professionals and the public about responding to biological and chemical terrorist incidents, as well as to nonterrorist incidents, such as epidemics and hazardous material incidents.

Spinal Cord Injury Centers

Spinal cord injury centers specialize in the medical, surgical, rehabilitative, and long-term follow-up care of the patient with a spinal cord injury.

Stroke Centers

Stroke centers specialize in diagnosing and treating diseases of the blood vessels of the brain. A stroke occurs when blood vessels to a part of the brain suddenly burst or become blocked. The staff at a stroke center works very quickly to determine the cause of the stroke and where it is located and give appropriate care.

Safety Priorities

1. Personal safety
2. Crew safety
3. Patient safety
4. Bystander safety

Roles of an EMT

The roles of an EMT include:

- Personal, crew, patient, and bystander safety
- Gaining access to the patient
- Performing a patient assessment to identify life-threatening conditions
- Continuing care through additional EMS resources
- Providing initial patient care based on the assessment findings
- Assisting with additional emergency care
- Documentation of the emergency per local and state requirements
- Acting as a public safety liaison

Responsibilities of an EMT

The responsibilities of an EMT include:

- Personal health and safety
- Maintaining a caring attitude and composure
- Maintaining a neat, clean, and professional appearance
- Maintaining up-to-date knowledge and skills
- Maintaining current knowledge of local, state, and national issues affecting EMS.

The Well-Being of the EMT

The Stages of Grief

- Grief is a normal response that helps a person cope with the loss of someone or something that had great meaning to him. Although grief is most often associated with death, any change of circumstance can cause us to go through this process.

- The 5 stages of grief are denial, anger, bargaining, depression, and acceptance. Remember that a person going through grief may skip a stage, go through more than 1 stage at the same time, or go through each stage more than once.

- Cultural factors will influence how a person experiences grief.

Death and Dying

Advance Directives and Do Not Resuscitate Orders

- Some patients may not want aggressive efforts aimed at reviving them when they are dying. These patients may have an advance directive or a Do Not Resuscitate (DNR) order.

- An advance directive is a legal document that details a person's healthcare wishes when he becomes unable to make decisions for himself.

- A DNR order is written by a physician. It instructs medical professionals not to provide medical care to a patient who has experienced a cardiac arrest.

Signs of Obvious Death

- The signs of obvious death include decapitation (beheading), putrefaction (decomposition), dependent lividity, and rigor mortis.
- If a person shows signs of obvious death, do not disturb the body or scene. The police or medical examiner will need to authorize removing the body.
- You should document the victim's position and his injuries. You should also document the conditions at the scene as well as statements of persons at the scene.

Recognizing Warning Signs of Stress
Physical Signs

- Increased heart rate
- Pounding/racing heart
- Elevated blood pressure
- Sweaty palms
- Tightness of the chest, neck, jaw, and back muscles
- Headache
- Diarrhea, constipation
- Trembling, twitching
- Stuttering and other speech difficulties
- Nausea, vomiting
- Sleep disturbances
- Fatigue
- Dryness of the mouth or throat
- Susceptibility to minor illness

Behavioral Signs

- Crying spells
- Hyperactivity or under-activity
- Changes in eating habits
- Increased substance use or abuse, including smoking, alcohol consumption, medications, and illegal substances
- Excessive humor or silence
- Violence, aggressive behavior
- Withdrawal
- Hostility
- Being prone to accidents
- Impatience

Mental Signs

- Inability to make decisions
- Forgetfulness
- Reduced creativity
- Lack of concentration
- Diminished productivity
- Lack of attention to detail
- Disorganized thoughts
- Lack of control or a need for too much control
- Inability to concentrate

Emotional Signs

- Irritability
- Angry outbursts
- Hostility
- Depression
- Jealousy
- Restlessness
- Withdrawal
- Anxiousness
- Diminished initiative
- Feelings of unreality or over-alertness
- Reduction of personal involvement with others
- Tendency to cry
- Being critical of others
- Nightmares
- Impatience
- Reduced self-esteem

Signs of Cumulative Stress

- Physical and emotional exhaustion
- A negative attitude toward others
- A disrespectful attitude toward patients
- Increased absences
- Emotional outbursts
- Decreased work performance

Infection Control
Methods of Disease Transmission

- Communicable diseases can be spread in different ways. Contact with drainage from an open sore is an example of direct contact. Germs can also be spread through indirect contact with contaminated materials or objects, such as needles, toys, drinking glasses, eating utensils, and bandages. Using gloves can help prevent the spread of disease from direct and indirect contact.

- Germs can also be transmitted in droplets suspended in the air through coughing, talking, and sneezing. Using a mask can help prevent the spread of infection from droplets. Using a mask that shields the eyes offers even better protection.

Classification of Communicable Diseases

Communicable diseases may be classified as airborne, bloodborne, foodborne, or sexually transmitted:

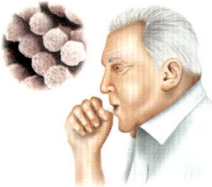

Airborne

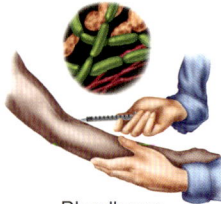

Bloodborne

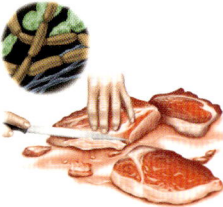

Foodborne

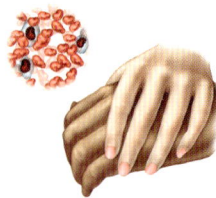

Sexually transmitted

- Airborne diseases are spread by droplets produced by coughing or sneezing. Examples include tuberculosis, measles, meningitis, rubella, smallpox, and chickenpox (varicella).
- Bloodborne diseases are spread by contact with the blood or body fluids of an infected person. Examples include hepatitis B virus, hepatitis C, human immunodeficiency virus (HIV), and syphilis.

- Foodborne diseases are spread by the improper handling of food or by poor personal hygiene. Examples include salmonella (food poisoning) and hepatitis A.
- Sexually transmitted diseases are spread by either blood or sexual contact. Examples include chlamydia, gonorrhea, and HIV.

Personal Protective Equipment

Personal Protective Equipment	Guidelines for Use
Gloves	Any situation in which there is potential for contacting blood or other body fluids
Gloves and chin-length plastic face shield (or mask and protective eyewear)	Any situation in which splashing or spattering of blood or other body fluids is likely
Gloves, chin-length plastic face shield (or mask and protective eyewear), and gown	Any situation in which splashing or spattering of blood or other body fluids is likely and clothing is likely to be soiled (such as childbirth, arterial bleeding)

Cleaning Equipment

- Cleaning is the process of washing a contaminated object with soap and water. An item must be cleaned before it is disinfected or sterilized. To clean equipment, begin by rinsing the item with cold water to remove obvious body fluid or tissue. Then wash the item with hot, soapy water. If the item has grooves or narrow spaces, use a stiff-bristled brush to clean it. Rinse it well with moderately hot water and then dry it. The item is now considered clean.

- Disinfecting is cleaning with chemical solutions such as alcohol or chlorine. These agents destroy some types of germs that may be left after washing. Depending on the type and degree of contamination, items such as stethoscopes, blood pressure cuffs, backboards, and splints usually need only cleaning followed by disinfection. Isopropyl (rubbing) alcohol is often used to disinfect surfaces. However, rubbing alcohol may discolor, swell, harden, and crack rubber and certain plastics after prolonged and repeated use. When chlorine bleach is used as a disinfectant, it must be diluted. A solution of 1 part bleach and 10 parts water or 1 part bleach and 100 parts water may be used. The solution used will depend on the amount of material (such as blood, mucus, or urine) present on the surface to be cleaned and disinfected. Many commercially available disinfectants are available. Follow the manufacturer's instructions to disinfect equipment.

- Sterilizing is a process that uses boiling water, radiation, gas, chemicals, or superheated steam to destroy all of the germs on an object. Reusable equipment that is inserted into a patient's body should always be sterilized.

Legal and Ethical Issues

Legal Duties of the EMT

- Provide for the well-being of the patient by giving emergency medical care as outlined in the scope of practice
- Provide the same standard of care as another EMT with similar training and experience in similar circumstances
- Before providing emergency care, make telephone or radio contact with your medical oversight authority (if required to do so)
- Follow standing orders and protocols approved by medical oversight or the local EMS system
- Follow instructions received from medical oversight

Ethical Responsibilities of the EMT

- Respond with respect to the physical and emotional needs of every patient
- Maintain mastery of skills
- Participate in continuing education and refresher programs
- Critically review your performance and seek improvement
- Report (written and verbal) honestly and accurately
- Respect confidentiality
- Work cooperatively and with respect for other emergency care professionals

Consent

- A competent patient must give you his consent (permission) before you can provide him with emergency care.
- Expressed consent is consent in which a patient gives specific permission for care and transport to be provided. Expressed consent may be given verbally, in writing, or nonverbally.
- Implied consent is consent assumed from a patient requiring emergency care who is mentally, physically, or emotionally unable to provide expressed consent.

Refusals

- Mentally competent adults have the right to refuse care and transport.
- As an EMT, you must make sure that the patient fully understands your explanation and the consequences of refusing treatment or transport. If a patient refuses treatment or transport, you must inform him of the following:
  - The nature of his illness or injury
  - The treatment that needs to be performed
  - The benefits of that treatment
  - The risks of not providing that treatment
  - Any alternatives to treatment
  - The dangers of refusing treatment (including transport)

- In high-risk situations in which the patient's injuries may not be obvious, you must contact medical direction or call ALS personnel to the scene to assess the patient.

Examples of High-Risk Refusals

- Abdominal pain
- Chest pain
- Electrical shock
- Foreign body ingestion
- Poisoning
- Pregnancy-related complaints
- Water-related incidents
- Falls >20 feet
- Head injury
- Vehicle rollovers
- High-speed auto crashes
- Auto-pedestrian or auto-bicycle injury with major impact (>5 mph)
- Pedestrian thrown or run over
- Motorcycle crash >20 mph or with the separation of the rider from the bike
- Pediatric patient with a vague medical complaint

Assault and Battery

- Assault is considered threatening to, attempting to, or causing a fear of offensive physical contact with a patient or other person.
- Battery is the unlawful touching of another person without consent.
- Because each state has its own definitions of assault and battery, you should check your local protocols concerning these terms.

Abandonment

Abandonment is terminating patient care without making sure that care will continue at the same level or higher. You can also be charged with abandonment if you stop patient care when the patient still needs and desires additional care.

Negligence

- When a healthcare professional is negligent, he fails to act as a reasonable, careful, similarly trained person would act under similar circumstances.
- Negligence includes the following 4 elements:
  1. The duty to act
  2. A breach of that duty
  3. Resulting injury or damages (physical or psychological)
  4. Proximate cause (the actions or inactions of the healthcare professional that caused the injury or damages)

The Human Body

Musculoskeletal System

The musculoskeletal system gives the human body its shape and ability to move and protects the major organs of the body. It consists of the skeletal system (bones) and the muscular system (muscles).

Respiratory System

- The respiratory system supplies oxygen from the air we breathe to the body's cells. It also removes carbon dioxide (a waste product of the body's cells) from the lungs when we breathe out.

- This system is made up of an upper and a lower airway. The upper airway includes the nose, the pharynx (throat), and the larynx (voice box). The lower airway consists of structures found mostly within the chest cavity, such as the trachea (windpipe) and the lungs.

Circulatory System

- The circulatory system is made up of the cardiovascular and lymphatic systems.

- This system has 3 main functions: (1) to deliver oxygen-rich blood and nutrients to body tissues, (2) to help maintain body temperature, and (3) to protect the body against infection.

- The cardiovascular system consists of the heart, blood, and blood vessels. The lymphatic system consists of lymph, lymph nodes, lymph vessels, tonsils, the spleen, and the thymus gland.

Nervous System

- The nervous system is a collection of specialized cells that transfer information to and from the brain. The 2 main functions of the nervous system are to control the voluntary (conscious) and involuntary (unconscious) activities of the body and to provide for higher mental function (such as thought and emotion).

- The nervous system has 2 divisions: (1) the central nervous system (CNS) and (2) the peripheral nervous system (PNS).

- The PNS has 2 divisions. The somatic (voluntary) division has receptors and nerves concerned with the external environment. It influences the activity of the musculoskeletal system. The autonomic (involuntary) division has receptors and nerves concerned with the internal environment. It controls the involuntary system of glands and smooth muscle and functions to maintain a steady state in the body.

- The autonomic division is divided into the sympathetic division and parasympathetic divisions. The sympathetic division mobilizes energy, particularly in stressful situations. This is called the "fight-or-flight" response. Its effects are widespread throughout the body. The parasympathetic division conserves and restores energy; its effects are localized in the body.

Integumentary System

- The integumentary system is made up of the skin, hair, nails, sweat glands, and oil (sebaceous) glands.
- The skin is the largest organ of the body. It protects the body from the environment, bacteria, and other organisms.

Digestive System

- The digestive system brings nutrients, water, and electrolytes into the body (ingestion). It chemically breaks down food into small parts so absorption can occur (digestion). It moves nutrients, water, and electrolytes into the circulatory system so they can be used by body cells (absorption). It also eliminates undigested waste (defecation).
- The primary organs of the digestive system are the mouth, pharynx, esophagus, stomach, small intestine, large intestine, rectum, and anal canal.
- The accessory organs are the teeth and tongue, salivary glands, liver, gallbladder, and pancreas.

Endocrine System

- The endocrine system is a system of glands that secrete chemicals (hormones) directly into the circulatory system. It works closely with the nervous system to maintain homeostasis.

Reproductive and Urinary Systems

- The reproductive system makes cells (sperm, eggs) that allow continuation of the human species.
- The urinary system produces and excretes urine from the body.

Baseline Vital Signs and SAMPLE History

Signs and Symptoms

- A sign is a medical or trauma condition of the patient that can be seen, heard, smelled, measured, or felt by the examiner. Examples of signs include unusual chest movement, bleeding, swelling, pale skin, and a fast pulse.
- A symptom is a condition described by the patient. Shortness of breath, nausea, abdominal pain, chills, chest pain, and dizziness are examples of symptoms.

Pulses

Central and Peripheral Pulses

Central Pulses	
Carotid	• Major artery of the neck • Supplies the head with blood • Pulsations can be found on either side of the neck • Avoid excess pressure in older adults • Never assess the carotid pulse on both sides of the neck at the same time
Femoral	• Located in the crease between the thigh and the pelvis • May require more pressure than other sites to be felt adequately

Peripheral Pulses	
Radial	• Located in the wrist at the base of the thumb • Used to assess circulation in the upper extremities • Should be checked first when assessing a responsive adult or child 1 year of age or older
Brachial	• Located on the inside of the upper arm, midway between the shoulder and the elbow • Used to assess circulation in the upper extremities • Always check this pulse in an infant
Posterior tibial	• Located just behind the ankle bone • Used to assess circulation in the lower extremities
Dorsalis pedis	• Located on the top surface of the foot • Used to assess circulation in the lower extremities

Pulse Rates

Count the number of beats for 30 seconds and multiply the number by 2 to determine the number of beats per minute. If the pulse is irregular, count it for 1 full minute.

Normal Pulse Rates at Rest

Life Stage	Age	Beats per Minute
Newborn	Birth to 1 month	120 to 160
Infant	1 to 12 months	80 to 140
Toddler	1 to 3 years	80 to 130
Preschooler	4 to 5 years	80 to 120
School-age child	6 to 12 years	70 to 110
Adolescent	13 to 18 years	60 to 100
Adult	18 years and older	60 to 100

Possible causes of a slow heart rate are:
- Good conditioning (a slow heart rate is normal in well-conditioned athletes)
- Heart problem, head injury, or hypothermia

Possible causes of a fast heart rate are:
- Normal response to the body's demand for more oxygen because of fever, fear, pain, anxiety, infection, shock, or exercise
- Drugs such as cocaine, some medications (such as epinephrine), or substances (such as caffeine and nicotine)

Pulse Quality

Pulse Strength

- Strong/full: normal pulse; easily felt
- Weak: hard to feel
- Thready: weak and fast

Pulse Rhythm

- Regular: Time elapses between beats are equal (regular and constant)
- Irregular: Beats are skipped or are unevenly spaced

Respiration

- Count respirations for 30 seconds and multiply the number by 2 to determine the rate for 1 minute. Count each rise and fall of the chest or abdomen as 1 respiration.
- If the patient's respirations are irregular or slow, count the rate for 1 full minute.
- Count an infant's respirations for 1 full minute.

Normal Respiratory Rates at Rest

Life Stage	Age	Breaths per Minute
Newborn	Birth to 1 month	30 to 50
Infant	1 to 12 months	20 to 40
Toddler	1 to 3 years	20 to 30

Preschooler	4 to 5 years	20 to 30
School-age child	6 to 12 years	16 to 30
Adolescent	13 to 18 years	12 to 20
Adult	18 years and older	12 to 20

Skin

Skin Finding	Possible Cause
Color	
Pale (white) skin	Shock, fright, anxiety
Cyanotic (blue) skin	Respiratory distress, airway obstruction, exposure to cold, blood vessel disease, shock
Mottled (patchy blue and white) skin	Shock, hypothermia, cardiac arrest
Jaundiced (yellow)	Liver or gallbladder problems
Flushed (red) skin	Heat exposure, late stages of carbon monoxide poisoning, allergic reaction, alcohol abuse, high blood pressure

Temperature and Condition (Moisture)	
Hot and dry or moist	Heat exposure
Warm and moist	Anxiety, warm environment, exercise
Cool and dry	Inadequate peripheral circulation, exposure to cold
Cool or cold and moist	Shock
Localized warmth	Infection, inflammation, or burn
Localized coolness	Poor arterial blood flow to a limb

Capillary Refill

- Assess capillary refill in infants and children 6 years of age or younger. Normal capillary refill time is less than 2 seconds.
- A capillary refill time of 3 to 5 seconds is said to be delayed. This may indicate poor perfusion or exposure to cool temperatures.
- A capillary refill time of more than 5 seconds is said to be markedly delayed and suggests shock.

Pupils

The pupils are normally equal in size, round, and equally reactive to light.

- *Size*. Dilated (very big) pupils in the presence of bright light may be due to trauma, fright, poisoning, eye medications, or glaucoma. Constricted (small) pupils in a darkened area may be caused by narcotics, treatment with eye drops, or a nervous system problem.

- *Equality*. In most patients, unequal pupils suggest a head injury, a stroke, the presence of an artificial eye, or cataract surgery on 1 eye.

- *Reactivity*. Reactivity refers to whether or not the pupils change in response to light. Normally, a light that is shined into the pupil of 1 eye will cause the pupils of both eyes to constrict. Nonreactive pupils do not change when exposed to light. This condition may occur because of medications or cardiac arrest. Unequally reactive pupils (1 pupil reacts but the other does not) may occur because of a head injury or stroke.

Blood Pressure

Normal Blood Pressure at Rest

Life Stage	Age	Systolic Pressure	Diastolic Pressure
Newborn	Birth to 1 month	74 to 100	50 to 68
Infant	1 to 12 months	84 to 106	56 to 70

Toddler	1 to 3 years	98 to 106	50 to 70
Preschooler	4 to 5 years	98 to 112	64 to 70
School-age child	6 to 12 years	104 to 124	64 to 80
Adolescent	13 to 18 years	118 to 132	70 to 82
Adult	18 years and older	100 to 119	60 to 79

Pulse Oximetry

- Pulse oximetry is a method of measuring the amount of oxygen saturated in the blood. Pulse oximetry is commonly referred to as *pulse ox.*

© *The McGraw-Hill Companies, Inc./Rick Brady, photographer*

- The oximeter calculates the amount of hemoglobin saturated with oxygen. This calculation is called *the saturation of peripheral oxygen* or S_pO_2. The oximeter displays this value as a percentage on its screen, as well as the patient's pulse rate.
- Pulse oximetry is used to detect and provide warnings about low levels of oxygen in the blood.
  —A reading between 96% and 100% generally indicates adequate oxygenation.
  —A reading between 91% and 95% suggests a mild lack of oxygen in the tissues (hypoxia).
  —A reading below 91% generally indicates severe hypoxia.

Indications

- Altered mental status
- Respiratory rate outside the normal range for age
- Increased work of breathing
- Respiratory or cardiac chief complaints
- History of respiratory difficulty or respiratory disease
- During delivery of supplemental oxygen
- During and after endotracheal intubation
- During transport of a sick or injured child

© The McGraw-Hill Companies, Inc./Rick Brady, photographer

End-Tidal Carbon Dioxide

An end-tidal carbon dioxide ($ETCO_2$) detector measures a person's exhaled carbon dioxide. Although an $ETCO_2$ detector is most often used to confirm the position of a tube that has been placed in a patient's trachea, some detectors can be used with oxygen delivery devices, such as a nasal cannula or bag-mask (BM) device.

Pain Assessment

- To assess pain in a child 3 years or older, use the Wong-Baker FACES Pain Rating Scale.
  - —This scale shows 6 cartoon faces ranging from a smiling face representing "no hurt" to a tearful, sad face representing "hurts worst."

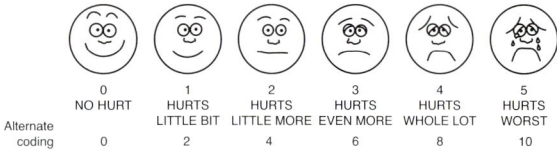

	0 NO HURT	1 HURTS LITTLE BIT	2 HURTS LITTLE MORE	3 HURTS EVEN MORE	4 HURTS WHOLE LOT	5 HURTS WORST
Alternate coding	0	2	4	6	8	10

From Hockenberry MJ, Wilson, D., Winkelstein, ML: Wong's Essentials of Pediatric Nursing, Ed. 7, St. Louis, 2005, p. 1259. Used with permission. Copyright, Mosby.

- Ask the patient to point to the face that best describes how he is feeling. Document the number indicated by the child.

SAMPLE History

A SAMPLE history includes the following:

*S*igns and symptoms

*A*llergies

*M*edications

(Pertinent) *P*ast medical history

*L*ast oral intake

*E*vents leading to the injury or illness

OPQRST

OPQRST is used to help identify the type and location of the patient's complaint:

Onset	"What were you doing when the problem started?"
Provocation/Palliation	"What makes the problem better or worse?"
Quality	"What does the pain feel like (dull, burning, sharp, stabbing, shooting, throbbing, pressure, or tearing)?"
Region/radiation	"Where is the pain?"
	"Is the pain in one area or does it move?"
	"Is the pain located in any other area?"
Severity	"On a scale of 0 to 10, with 0 being no pain and 10 being the worst, what number would you give your pain or discomfort?"
Time	"How long ago did the problem/discomfort begin?"
	"Have you ever had this pain before?" "When? How long did it last?"

Lifting and Moving Patients

Safe Lifting

Safe lifting means keeping your back aligned as vertically as possible, using your leg strength, and maintaining your center of balance while lifting. Follow these important rules to prevent injury when lifting:

- Consider the weight of the patient and the need for additional help.
- Know your physical ability and limitations.
- Plan how you will move the patient and where you will move him. Consider using a sturdy chair or commercially made stair chair when transporting patients down stairs.
- Mentally picture the patient's final position and work backward to the patient's current position. This helps prevent arms from getting crossed and bodies from becoming twisted during the actual move.
- Make sure your path is clear of obstructions.
- When working with others, determine in advance who will direct the move. *One* person (usually the person at the patient's head) must assume responsibility for directing the actions of the others. "On my count, lift on 3: 1, 2, 3." "On my count, turn on 3: 1, 2, 3." Agree in advance that if anyone involved in the move says "No," the move will immediately be stopped. The person stopping the move must state what needs to be done in order to complete the move.

- Position your feet a comfortable distance apart (usually a shoulder's width) on a firm surface. Wear proper footwear to protect your feet and maintain a firm footing.
- Tense the muscles of your abdomen and buttocks before lifting. This helps relieve the stress on your back muscles.
- Bend at your knees and hips, not your waist, keeping your back straight. All movement in the lift comes from your *legs*.
- Use your legs to lift, not your back. Your legs are much stronger than your back.
- Lift by using a smooth, continuous motion. *Do not jerk or twist* when lifting.
- Keep the patient's weight as close to you as possible. ("Hug the load.") This moves your center of gravity closer to the patient, helps maintain balance, and reduces muscle strain.
- When possible, move forward rather than backward.
- Walk slowly, using short steps.
- Look where you are going.
- Move slowly, communicating clearly and frequently with other EMS personnel and the patient throughout the move.

Safe Reaching

To avoid injury when reaching, following these important rules:

- Keep your back straight.
- Avoid stretching or leaning back from your waist (hyperextending) when reaching overhead. Lean from your hips.
- Avoid twisting while reaching.
- Avoid reaching more than 15-20 inches in front of your body to grasp an object.
- Avoid situations in which prolonged (more than a minute) strenuous effort is needed.

Safe Pushing and Pulling

To avoid injury when pushing and pulling, follow these guidelines:

- Push, rather than pull, whenever possible.
- Keep your back straight.
- Avoid twisting or jerking when pushing or pulling an object.
- Push at a level between your waist and shoulders.
- When the patient or object is below your waist, kneel to push or pull.
- When pulling, avoid reaching more than 15-20 inches in front of your body. Change your position (move back another 15-20 inches) when your hands have reached the front of your body.

- Keep the line of pull through the center of your body by bending your knees.
- Keep the weight close to your body.
- Keep your elbows bent with your arms close to your sides.
- If possible, avoid pushing or pulling from an overhead position.

Airway and Breathing

Airway

Opening the Airway

- The head tilt–chin lift maneuver is used to open the airway if trauma to the head or neck is not suspected.

- When trauma to the head or neck of an unresponsive patient is suspected, you should use the jaw thrust without head tilt (also called the *jaw thrust without head extension maneuver*) to open the patient's airway. However, use a head tilt–chin lift maneuver if the jaw thrust does not open the airway. This method of opening the airway is effective, but it is less effective than the head tilt–chin lift and is more tiring. Because the head tilt-chin lift requires the use of both hands, a second rescuer will be needed if the patient requires ventilation.

Clearing the Airway

If a patient's airway is obstructed, you must clear it. The 3 primary ways of clearing the airway of an unresponsive patient are with the recovery position, finger sweeps, and suctioning.

- You can use the recovery position as the first step in maintaining an open airway in an unresponsive patient. This position involves positioning a patient on his side. Remember not to place a patient with a known or suspected spinal injury in the recovery position.

- If you see foreign material in the patient's mouth, you must remove it immediately. If foreign material is seen in an unresponsive patient's upper airway, a finger sweep may be used to remove it.

- A "blind" finger sweep is performed without first seeing foreign material in the airway. Blind finger sweeps should *never* be performed. Doing so may cause the object to become further lodged in the patient's throat.

- Always have suction equipment with arm's reach when you are managing a patient's airway or assisting a patient's breathing. Suctioning is a procedure used to vacuum vomitus, saliva, blood, food particles, and other material from the patient's airway.

- Apply suction while moving the tip of the catheter from side to side as you withdraw it from the patient's mouth. Because you are removing air (oxygen) from the patient when suctioning, do not suction an adult for more than 15 seconds at a time. When suctioning an infant or child, do not apply suction for more than 10 seconds at a time.

Airway Adjuncts

After you have opened a patient's airway, you may need to use an airway adjunct to keep it open. After the airway adjunct is inserted, the proper head position must be maintained while the device is in place.

- An oral airway is a device that is used only in unresponsive patients without a gag reflex. It is inserted into the patient's mouth and used to keep the tongue away from the back of the throat.
- A nasal airway is a device that is placed in the patient's nose. It keeps the patient's tongue from blocking the upper airway. It also allows air to flow from the hole in the device down into the patient's lower airway.

Breathing

After making sure that the patient's airway is open, you must check for breathing. If the patient is breathing, you must determine whether the patient is breathing adequately or inadequately. You must also be able to recognize the sounds of noisy breathing, which include stridor, snoring, wheezing, gurgling, and crowing.

Signs of Adequate Breathing

- Breathing is quiet and effortless and does not involve the use of accessory muscles
- Respiratory rate is within normal limits for the patient's age
- Respiratory rhythm is regular, with symmetrical chest expansion
- Respiratory depth is adequate
- Skin color is normal; skin is warm and dry to the touch

Signs of Inadequate Breathing

- Respiratory rate is outside normal ranges for the patient's age
- Breathing pattern is irregular
- Breath sounds are diminished or absent
- Chest expansion is unequal or inadequate
- Work of breathing (effort) is increased
- Respiratory depth is inadequate (shallow respirations)
- Skin is pale, cyanotic (blue), cool, and clammy

Abnormal Respiratory Sounds

Respiratory Sound	Description	Possible Cause
Stridor	Harsh, high-pitched sound (like the bark of a seal); usually heard during inhalation	Severe upper airway obstruction, croup
Snoring	Noisy breathing through the mouth and nose	Partial upper airway obstruction by the tongue

Wheezing	High-pitched whistling sound heard on inhalation or exhalation	Air movement through narrowed airway passages; asthma, anaphylaxis
Gurgling	Wet sound heard as air passes through moist secretions in the airway	Liquid or semi-solid material in the patient's upper airway
Crowing	Long, high-pitched sound heard on inhalation	Croup

Respiratory Distress, Respiratory Failure, and Respiratory Arrest

A patient who is showing signs of respiratory distress will often progress to respiratory failure if you do not work quickly to relieve his symptoms.

- Respiratory distress is increased work of breathing (respiratory effort). A patient who has signs and symptoms of inadequate breathing must be considered to be experiencing respiratory distress.

- In respiratory failure, there is inadequate blood oxygenation and/or ventilation to meet the demands of body tissues. A patient in respiratory failure looks very sick and often very tired. Signs of greatly increased work of breathing are usually present. The patient's skin may appear pale, mottled, or blue.

- If respiratory failure is not corrected, it will usually progress to respiratory arrest. If not corrected, respiratory arrest will, in turn, rapidly lead to cardiac arrest. Agonal breathing is slow and shallow breathing that is sometimes seen just before the onset of respiratory arrest.

- Other signs and symptoms of respiratory arrest include the following:

  —Unresponsiveness

  —No air movement from the mouth or nose

  —No chest rise and fall

  —Changes in skin color as a result of a lack of oxygen

- Think of respiratory distress, failure, and arrest as increasing levels of severity of a respiratory problem. If you do not move quickly to resolve it, the respiratory problem will also become a cardiac problem.

How to Ventilate

- If your patient's breathing is inadequate or absent, you will need to assist the patient by forcing air into the patient's lungs during inspiration. This action is called *positive-pressure ventilation.* Mouth-to-mask ventilation, mouth-to-barrier ventilation, mouth-to-mouth ventilation, and BM ventilation are methods used to deliver positive-pressure ventilation.

- If positive-pressure ventilation is performed too rapidly or with too much volume, air can enter the stomach. When pressure is applied to the cricoid cartilage, the trachea is pushed backward and the esophagus is compressed (closed) against the cervical vertebrae. This compression helps decrease the amount of air entering the stomach during positive-pressure ventilation, which reduces the likelihood of vomiting and aspiration. Cricoid pressure (also called the *Sellick maneuver*) should be used only in unresponsive patients. It is usually applied by a third person during positive-pressure ventilation.

- A flow-restricted, oxygen-powered ventilation device is used to give positive-pressure ventilation with 100% oxygen. It can be attached to a face mask, tracheal tube, or tracheostomy tube.

- A BM device can be used to assist ventilations in a patient with inadequate breathing, but it is more commonly used to ventilate a nonbreathing patient.
  —When a BM is not connected to supplemental oxygen, 21% oxygen (room air) is delivered to the patient.

21% O_2

Room air

21% O_2

  —If a BM is connected to supplemental oxygen set at a flow rate of 15 L/min but no reservoir is used, about 40-60% oxygen can be delivered to the patient, provided there is a good face-to-mask seal.

40–60% O_2

100% O_2 (15L/min)

Room air (21% O_2)

40–60% O_2

—If the BM is connected to supplemental oxygen at a flow rate of 15 L/min and a reservoir is present on the bag, about 90-100% oxygen can be delivered to the patient, provided there is a good face-to-mask seal.

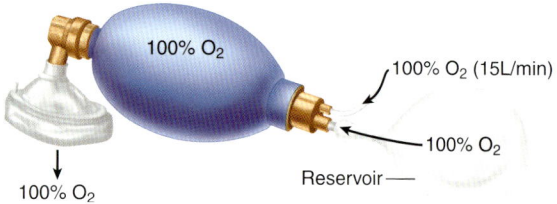

100% O_2

100% O_2 (15L/min)

100% O_2

Reservoir

100% O_2

Rates for Positive-Pressure Ventilation

Patient	Breaths/Minute	Length of Each Breath
Adult	10 to 12 (1 breath every 5 to 6 seconds)	1 second
Infant/Child	12 to 20 (1 breath every 3 to 5 seconds)	1 second
Newborn	40 to 60 (1 breath every 1 to 1.5 seconds)	1 second

Oxygen Cylinders

Cylinder Type	Amount of Oxygen in Liters
Portable	
D	425
Jumbo D	640
E	680
Onboard	
M	3450
G	5300
H	6900

Oxygen Delivery Devices

- The 2 most common oxygen delivery devices are the nonrebreather (NRB) mask and the nasal cannula.

  —In most situations, a NRB mask is the preferred method of oxygen delivery in the field for a patient who is breathing adequately. At 15 L/min, the oxygen concentration delivered is about 90%.

  —The use of a nasal cannula requires a breathing patient. A nasal cannula can deliver an oxygen concentration of 25-45% at 1-6 L/min. Flow rates of more than 6 L/min are irritating to the nasal passages.

Scene Size-Up

Components of Scene Size-Up

- Body substance isolation (BSI) precautions
- Evaluation of scene safety
- Determining the mechanism of injury (MOI) (including considerations for stabilization of the spine) or the nature of the patient's illness
- Determining the total number of patients
- Determining the need for additional resources

Patient Assessment

Components of Patient Assessment

- The primary survey is a rapid assessment to find and treat all immediate life-threatening conditions. You must perform a primary survey on *every* patient.

- The secondary survey is a physical examination performed to discover medical conditions and/or injuries that were not identified in the primary survey. During this phase of the patient assessment, you will also obtain vital signs, reassess changes in the patient's condition, and determine the patient's chief complaint, history of present illness, and significant past medical history.

- A general impression (also called a *first impression*) is an "across-the-room" assessment. You can complete it in 60 seconds or less. The purpose of forming a general impression is to decide if the patient looks "sick" or "not sick." If the patient looks sick, you must act quickly. Base your general impression of a patient on 3 main areas: (1) appearance, (2) breathing, and (3) circulation.

- After forming a general impression, begin the primary survey by assessing the patient's airway and level of responsiveness. Assessment of a patient's airway and level of responsiveness occur

PATIENT ASSESSMENT

Initial Assessment

Scene Size-Up

Primary Survey	Secondary Survey
General Impression: Appearance (Work of) Breathing Circulation	Vital signs
Airway + Level of responsiveness Cervical spine protection	Focused history (SAMPLE, OPQRST)
Breathing (Ventilation)	Head-to-toe (or focused) physical exam
Circulation (Perfusion)	
Disability (Mini-neurological exam)	
Expose	

Ongoing Assessment

at the same time. A patient's mental status is "graded" by using a scale called the *AVPU scale:*

—A = **A**lert

—V = Responds to **V**erbal stimuli

—P = Responds to **P**ainful stimuli

—U = **U**nresponsive

- A patient who is oriented to person, place, time, and event is said to be "alert and oriented × ('times') 4" or "A and O × 4." Assessing the mental status of a child older than 3 years of age is the same as that of an adult.

- For trauma patients or unresponsive patients with an unknown nature of illness, take spinal precautions. Spinal precautions are used to stabilize the head, neck, and back in a neutral position. This stabilization is done to minimize movement that could cause injury to the spinal cord.

- After making sure that the patient's airway is open, assess the patient's breathing to determine if breathing is adequate or inadequate. If the patient is unresponsive and breathing is inadequate or if the patient is not breathing, begin positive-pressure ventilation using a pocket mask, mouth-to-barrier device, or BM device.

- Assessment of circulation involves evaluating for signs of obvious bleeding; central and peripheral pulses; skin color, temperature, and condition; and capillary refill (in children 6 years of age or younger). Look from the patient's head to toes for signs of significant external bleeding. Control major bleeding, if present.

- Altered mental status means a change in a patient's level of awareness. Altered mental status is also called an *altered level of consciousness* (ALOC). A patient who has an altered mental status is at risk of an airway obstruction. Most EMS systems use the Glasgow Coma Scale (GCS) during the disability phase of the primary survey to obtain a more detailed assessment of the patient's neurological status. Three categories are assessed with the GCS: (1) eye opening, (2) verbal response, and (3) motor response.
- Expose pertinent areas of the patient's body for examination. Factors that you must consider when exposing the patient include protecting the patient's modesty, the presence of bystanders, and environment/weather conditions.
- Determine if the patient requires on-scene stabilization or immediate transport ("load and go" situations) with additional emergency care en route to a hospital.
- The secondary survey is patient, situation, and time dependent. A secondary survey (head-to-toe assessment) should be performed in the following situations:

   —Trauma patients with a significant MOI

   —Trauma patients with an unknown or unclear MOI

   —Trauma patients with an injury to more than 1 area of the body

   —All unresponsive patients

—All patients with an altered mental status

—Some responsive medical patients, on the basis of history and focused physical examination findings

- A quick secondary survey of a trauma patient with a significant MOI is called a *rapid trauma assessment*. A significant MOI is one that is likely to produce serious injury.

- A quick secondary survey of a medical patient who is unresponsive or has an altered mental status is called a *rapid medical assessment*.

- The phrase *focused physical examination* is used to describe an assessment of specific body areas that relate to the patient's illness or injury. The procedure for performing a secondary survey is the same for trauma and medical patients. However, the physical findings that you are looking for and discover may have a different meaning depending on whether the patient is a trauma or medical patient.

- DCAP-BTLS is a helpful memory aid to remember what to look and feel for during the physical exam:

  Deformities

  Contusions (bruises)

  Abrasions (scrapes)

  Punctures/penetrations

  Burns

  Tenderness

  Lacerations (cuts)

  Swelling

- Remember to take 2 or more sets of vital signs. Doing so will allow you to note changes (trends) in the patient's condition and response to treatment. Reassess and record vital signs at least every 5 minutes in an unstable patient and at least every 15 minutes in a stable patient.
- The conclusion you reach about what is wrong with your patient is called a *field impression.*
- The history of the present illness is a chronological record of the reason a patient is seeking medical assistance. It includes the patient's chief complaint and the patient's answers to questions about the circumstances that led up to the request for medical help. The chief complaint is the reason why the patient called for assistance.
- An ongoing assessment consists of 4 main areas:
  1. Repeating the primary survey
  2. Reassessing vital signs
  3. Repeating the focused assessment
  4. Reevaluating emergency care
- An ongoing assessment should be performed on every patient. It is performed after the secondary survey, if one is performed. In some situations, the patient's condition may prevent performance of a secondary survey. An ongoing assessment is usually performed en route to the receiving facility. However, if transport is delayed, the ongoing assessment should be performed on the scene.
- Repeat the ongoing assessment at least every 15 minutes for a stable patient and every 5 minutes for an unstable patient.

Communications

Federal Communications Commission

- The Federal Communications Commission is the U.S. government agency responsible for the development and enforcement of rules and regulations pertaining to radio transmissions.

Radio Frequencies

- Very high frequency (VHF) radio frequencies can be subdivided into low-band and high-band. Low-band frequencies generally have a greater range than high-band VHF frequencies. Radio waves in the low-band frequency range bend and follow the curvature of the earth, allowing radio transmission over long distances. Radio waves in the high-band frequency range travel in a straight line. This straight-line quality means that the radio wave is easily blocked by topography such as a hill, mountain, or large building.

- Ultra-high frequency (UHF) radio waves travel in a straight line but do have an ability to reflect or bounce around buildings. 800-Megahertz frequencies are UHF radio signals that use computer technology to make transmissions more secure than the other types of radio transmission.

Documentation

Characteristics of Good Documentation

- Good documentation is complete, clear, concise, objective, timely, accurate, and legible.

Uses of the Prehospital Care Report

- Continuity of care. The Prehospital Care Report (PCR) may be used by receiving facility staff to help determine the direction of treatment following the EMS treatments given.
- Legal document. Good documentation reflects the emergency medical care provided, status of the patient on arrival at the scene, and any changes upon arrival at the receiving facility.
- Education and research. The PCR can be used to show proper documentation and how to handle unusual or uncommon situations, as well as identify training needs for the EMS providers.
- Administrative. The PCR is used for billing and EMS service statistics.
- Quality management. Completed reports are typically evaluated for adequacy of documentation, compliance with local rules and regulations, compliance with agency documentation standards, and appropriateness of medical care.

Error Correction

- When a documentation error occurs, do not try to cover it up. Instead, document what did or did not happen, time, date, and initial your entry.

Pharmacology

Drug Names

- A drug's chemical name is a description of its composition and molecular structure.
- The generic name (also called the *nonproprietary name*) is the name given to a drug by the company that first manufactures it.
- A drug's trade name is also known as its *brand name* or *proprietary name*.

Drug Effects

- A local effect of a drug usually occurs only in a limited part of the body (usually at the site of drug application).
- Drugs with systemic effects are absorbed into the bloodstream and distributed throughout the body.

Drug Administration

Before giving a drug, you must know the following:

- The drug's mechanism of action: the desired effects the drug should have on the patient

- Indications for the drug's use, including the most common uses of the drug in treating a specific illness

- Contraindications: situations in which the drug should not be used because it may cause harm to the patient or offer no possibility of improving the patient's condition or illness

- The correct dose (amount) of the drug to be given

- The proper route by which the drug is given

- Side effects: the actions of a drug other than those desired. Some side effects may be predictable.

Medications that are typically carried on the EMS unit and may be given by EMTs include activated charcoal, oral glucose, and oxygen. Some EMS systems also include aspirin and naloxone.

Medications an EMT can assist a patient in taking with approval by medical direction include a prescribed inhaler, nitroglycerin, and an epinephrine auto-injector.

Routes of Drug Administration

- The oral route of drug administration is used infrequently in the prehospital setting. Commonly used oral dosage forms include liquids, tablets, and capsules. Activated charcoal may be given by this route. Patients who are unresponsive, uncooperative, have no gag reflex, or are vomiting should not be given drugs orally.

- Drugs administered by the buccal route are placed in the mouth against the mucous membranes of the cheek until the drug is dissolved. The drug may act locally on the mucous membranes of the mouth or systemically when swallowed in the saliva. Buccal drugs are rapidly absorbed into the bloodstream. Oral glucose may be given by this route.

- Sublingual drugs are given under the tongue. The drug must remain under the tongue until it is dissolved and absorbed. The drug is absorbed rapidly into the bloodstream because of the rich blood supply under the tongue. Nitroglycerin may be given by this route.

- Drugs given by the inhalation route have a rapid onset of action because of the large surface area and blood supply of the lungs. To make sure that normal gas exchange of oxygen and carbon dioxide is continuous in the lungs, drugs given by inhalation must be in the form of a gas (such as oxygen) or fine mist (such as an aerosol). Oxygen is given for its systemic effects. A metered-dose inhaler (MDI) such as albuterol is given for its localized effect on the lungs.

- Drugs given by the subcutaneous (SubQ) route are given by means of a needle inserted underneath the skin into the subcutaneous tissue. The onset of action of SubQ drugs is faster than the oral route but slower than the intramuscular route. Absorption is delayed in circulatory collapse, such as shock. Only a small volume of drug can be given by this route.
- When a drug is given by the intramuscular route, a medication in a liquid form is injected into a large mass of skeletal muscle. The onset of action is faster than the SubQ route because of the muscle's blood supply and large absorbing surface. Epinephrine is an example of a drug that may be given by this route.

General Guidelines

Before giving a drug, use the 5 rights of drug administration.

1. *Right patient.* If assisting a patient in taking his own medication, make sure that the medication is prescribed for *that* patient.
2. *Right drug.* Select the right medication. Only use medications that are in a clearly labeled container. If the label is unclear or blurred, do not give the drug. Carefully read the label and check it 3 times before administering: (1) when removing the drug from the drug box, (2) when preparing the drug for administration, and (3) before actually giving the drug to the patient. Check the drug's expiration date.

3. *Right dose*. Check and recheck the dose ordered against the dose to be given.
4. *Right route*. You must know the route(s) by which a drug is to be given.
5. *Right time* (*frequency*). Although many drugs are ordered for 1-time administration, some may be repeated. Determine from medical direction the frequency with which a drug may be given.

Respiratory Emergencies

Levels of Respiratory Distress

No Breathing Difficulty

- The patient appears relaxed and denies shortness of breath.
- The patient's breathing is quiet and unlabored.
- The patient is able to speak in full sentences without pausing to catch his breath.
- The patient's breathing is regular and at a rate within normal limits for his age.
- The patient's breathing pattern is smooth and regular. There is equal rise and fall of the chest with each breath. The patient may have occasional sighing respirations.
- The patient's depth of breathing (tidal volume) is adequate.
- The color of the patient's skin and the mucous membranes of his mouth are normal.

Mild Breathing Difficulty

- The patient may be hypoxic but can move an adequate amount of air.
- The patient's heart rate and respiratory rate may be increased.
- The patient is alert and can answer your questions in complete sentences.

Moderate Breathing Difficulty

- The patient may be hypoxic, but he can still move an adequate amount of air (although his tidal volume may be decreased).
- The patient may be awake but is restless and irritable.
- The patient has an increased heart rate and respiratory rate.
- The patient has difficulty answering questions and is unable to speak in complete sentences.

Severe Breathing Difficulty

- The patient may be sleepy or unresponsive.
- The patient may have been wild and combative but now appears quiet. This is a sign of respiratory failure. The patient is wearing out.
- If the patient is responsive, he may be unable to speak or may only be able to speak in short phrases of 1 to 2 words.
- The patient may assume a tripod position and may need support to maintain a sitting position as he tires.
- The patient's breathing rate may initially be rapid with periods of slow breathing. As he tires and his condition worsens, his breathing rate will slow and then become agonal (gasping) respirations.
- As the patient's breathing muscles tire, his breathing becomes shallow.
- The patient's skin may appear blue or mottled despite having been given oxygen.

Comparison of Croup and Epiglottitis

	Croup	Epiglottitis
Age	6 months to 3 years	3 to 7 years
Cause	Viral	Bacterial
Onset	Gradual	Sudden
Signs/Symptoms	• Stridor • Barking cough • Hoarse voice • Low-grade fever (usually <102.2°F)	• Stridor • Restlessness • Sore throat, drooling • Muffled voice • High fever (usually 102°F to 104°F) • Tripod position, unwilling to lie down • Difficulty swallowing • Dyspnea

Prescribed Metered-Dose Inhaler

Generic (Trade) name	• albuterol (Proventil, Ventolin) • isoetharine (Bronkosol) • metaproterenol (Alupent, Metaprel) • fluticasone and salmeterol (Advair)
Mechanism of action	• Dilates bronchioles, reducing airway resistance

Indications	An EMT can assist a patient in taking a prescribed inhaler if *all* of the following criteria are met: • The patient has signs and symptoms of a respiratory emergency. • The patient has a physician-prescribed handheld inhaler. • There are no contraindications to giving the medication. • The EMT has specific authorization by medical direction.
Dosage	An MDI automatically delivers a specific dose of medication each time it is activated. The usual dosage is 2 puffs every 3 to 4 hours as needed for shortness of breath associated with asthma and COPD. The number of inhalations is based on medical direction's order or the patient's physician order.
Side effects	• Increased heart rate • Shaking or tremors • Nervousness
Contrain-dications	• Medical direction does not give permission. • Patient is unable to use the device • Inhaler is not prescribed for the patient. • Patient has already met maximum prescribed dose before EMT arrival.

Cardiovascular Emergencies

Heart Disease Risk Factors

Modifiable Factors	Non-modifiable Factors	Contributing Factors
Diabetes mellitus	Family history	Stress
High blood pressure	Gender	Depression
Elevated blood cholesterol	Race	Heavy alcohol intake (3 or more drinks per day)
Tobacco smoke	Increasing age	
Lack of exercise		
Obesity		

Angina Pectoris: Possible Triggers

- Physical exertion
- Emotional upset
- Eating a heavy meal
- Exposure to extreme hot or cold temperatures
- Cigarette smoking

- Sexual activity
- Stimulants, such as caffeine or cocaine

Typical Heart Attack: Signs and Symptoms

- Uncomfortable squeezing, ache, dull pressure, or pain in the center of the chest lasting more than a few minutes
- Discomfort in one or both arms, the back, neck, jaw, or stomach
- Anxiety, dizziness, irritability
- Abnormal pulse rate (may be irregular)
- Abnormal blood pressure
- Nausea, vomiting
- Lightheadedness
- Fainting or near-fainting
- Breaking out in a cold sweat
- Weakness
- Shortness of breath
- Difficulty breathing (dyspnea)
- Palpitations
- Feeling of impending doom

Atypical Heart Attack: Signs and Symptoms

Older Adults	Diabetic Individuals	Women
Unexplained new-onset or worsened difficulty of breathing with exertion	Change in mental status	Pain or discomfort in the chest, arms, back, shoulders, neck, jaw, or stomach
Unexplained nausea, vomiting	Weakness	Anxiety, dizziness
Sweating	Fainting	Shortness of breath
Unexplained tiredness	Lightheadedness	Weakness
Change in mental status	Shoulder/back pain	Unusual tiredness
Weakness		Cold sweats
Fainting		Nausea, vomiting
Abdominal discomfort		

Aspirin

Generic name	acetylsalicylic acid
Trade name	Bayer, Ecotrin, Empirin
Mechanism of action	Blocks a part of the clotting process in the bloodstream and may reduce the risk of a heart attack
Indications	Chest pain or discomfort that is suspected to be of cardiac origin
Dosage (adult)	Two to four 81-mg tablets (baby aspirin), chewed and swallowed
Side effects	• Rapid pulse • Dizziness • Flushing • Nausea, vomiting • Gastrointestinal bleeding
Contraindications	• Known allergy or sensitivity to aspirin • Bleeding ulcer or bleeding disorders • Stroke • Children and adolescents

Nitroglycerin

Generic name	nitroglycerin
Trade name	Nitrostat, Nitrobid, Nitrolingual, Nitroglycerin Spray
Mechanism of action	• Relaxes blood vessels, thus increasing the flow of oxygenated blood to the heart muscle • Decreases the workload of the heart
Indications	An EMT can assist a patient in taking nitroglycerin if *all* of the following criteria are met: • The patient has signs and symptoms of chest discomfort suspected to be of cardiac origin. • The patient has physician-prescribed sublingual tablets or spray. • There are no contraindications to giving nitroglycerin. • The EMT has specific authorization by medical direction.

Dosage	Dosage is 1 tablet or 1 spray under the tongue. This dose may be repeated in 3 to 5 minutes (maximum of 3 doses) if: • The patient experiences no relief • The patient's systolic blood pressure remains above 100 mm Hg • The patient's heart rate remains between 50 and 100 beats/min • There are no other contraindications, and • The EMT is authorized by medical direction to give another dose of the medication.
Side effects	Hypotension is a common and significant side effect. Other side effects include tachycardia, bradycardia, headache, palpitations, and fainting.
Contraindications	• No permission from medical direction • Medication not prescribed for the patient

	• Maximum prescribed dose already taken by patient before EMT arrival
	• Hypotension or blood pressure < 100 mm Hg systolic
	• Heart rate < 50 beats/min or > 100 beats/min
	• Head injury (recent) or stroke (recent)
	• Infants and children
	• Patient who has taken a medication for erectile dysfunction within the last 24-48 hours

Chain of Survival

1. Early access (recognition of an emergency and calling 9-1-1)
2. Early cardiopulmonary resuscitation (CPR)
3. Early defibrillation (the delivery of an electrical shock to the heart)
4. Early advanced cardiac life support (ACLS)

Cardiac Arrest

If you arrive on the scene of a cardiac arrest, begin CPR if:

- A DNR order is not present
- There are no signs of obvious death

- A DNR order is present but the DNR documentation is unclear
- A DNR order is present but you are not sure the order is valid

If you arrive on the scene of a cardiac arrest and a DNR order is present:

- Make sure the form clearly identifies the person to whom the DNR applies
- Make sure the patient is the person referred to in the DNR document
- Make sure the document is of the correct type approved by your state and local authorities

CPR Guidelines

	Adult	Child	Infant
Patient Age	More than 12 to 14 years	1 to 12 to 14 years	Under 1 year
Rescue Breaths	About 10-12 breaths/min 1 breath every 5-6 seconds	About 12-20 breaths/min 1 breath every 3-5 seconds	About 12-20 breaths/min 1 breath every 3-5 seconds

Location of Pulse Check	Carotid	Carotid	Brachial
Method of Chest Compressions	Heel of 1 hand, other hand on top	Heel of 1 hand or same as for adult	2 fingers (1 rescuer) or 2 thumbs with the fingers of both hands encircling the chest (2 rescuers)
Depth of Chest Compressions	1½ to 2 inches	⅓ to ½ the chest depth	⅓ to ½ the chest depth
Rate of Chest Compressions	About 100/min		
Ratio of Chest Compressions to Rescue Breaths (One Cycle)	1 or 2 rescuers: 30 compressions to 2 breaths (30:2)	1 rescuer: 30 compressions to 2 breaths (30:2) 2 rescuers: 15 compressions to 2 breaths (15:2)	1 rescuer: 30 compressions to 2 breaths (30:2) 2 rescuers: 15 compressions to 2 breaths (15:2)

When to Stop CPR

You should stop CPR only if:

- Effective breathing and circulation have returned
- The scene becomes unsafe
- You are too exhausted to continue
- You transfer patient care to a healthcare professional with equal or higher certification
- A physician assumes responsibility for the patient

Using an AED

Use the following steps to operate an automatic external defibrillator (AED):

1. Power
2. Pads
3. Analyze
4. Shock

Diabetes and Altered Mental Status

Altered Mental Status: Common Causes

A-E-I-O-U TIPPS

- *A*lcohol, Abuse
- *E*pilepsy (seizures)
- *I*nsulin (diabetic emergency)
- *O*verdose, (lack of) oxygen (hypoxia)
- *U*remia (kidney failure)
- *T*rauma (head injury), Temperature (fever, heat- or cold-related emergency)
- *I*nfection
- *P*sychiatric conditions
- *P*oisoning (including drugs and alcohol)
- *S*hock, Stroke

Major Types of Diabetes Mellitus

Diabetes Type	Other Names	Possible Causes
Type 1	Insulin-dependent diabetes mellitus Juvenile diabetes	Usually unknown Viral infection Injury to pancreas Immune system disorder
Type 2	Non-insulin-dependent diabetes mellitus Adult-onset diabetes	Insulin resistance and relative insulin shortage

Gestational	Diabetes during pregnancy	Changes in body metabolism caused by pregnancy

Hypoglycemia and Hyperglycemia

	Hypoglycemia	Hyperglycemia
Onset	Sudden (minutes to hours)	Gradual (hours to days)
Signs and symptoms	Altered mental status (varies from nervousness to coma) Early signs • Sweating • Palpitations • Increased heart rate • Tremors • Pale color • Hunger • Headache • Nervousness	Altered mental status (varies from drowsiness to coma) Rapid, deep breathing (Kussmaul respirations) Sweet or fruity (acetone) breath odor Loss of appetite Thirst Dry skin Abdominal pain Nausea and/or vomiting Increased heart rate

	Later signs	Normal or slightly decreased blood pressure
	• Confusion, combativeness, irritability, difficulty concentrating	Weakness
	• Tiredness	
	• Staggering walk	
	• Visual disturbances	
	• Cool, pale, clammy skin	
	• Fainting	
	• Seizures	
	• Coma	

Blood Glucose Testing: Indications

1. Unresponsive patient, cause unknown (any age group, including trauma)

2. Known diabetic patient with any of the following signs and symptoms:

   • Altered mental status (confusion, change in usual behavior)

   • Unresponsive

   • Slurred speech

   • Cold and clammy skin or hot, dry skin/mucous membranes

- Pale or flushed color
- Sweating
- Headache, dizziness
- Palpitations and/or abnormal heart rhythm seen on heart monitor
- Visual disturbances
- Shakiness or statement that he "feels funny"
- Excessive urination/thirst
- Acetone (fruity) breath
- Rapid, deep breathing (Kussmaul respirations)
- Seizures

3. Patients with altered mental status, cause unknown (including trauma), especially if showing signs and symptoms listed previously

4. Special situations
   - Infant or child having seizures or an altered mental status
   - Pregnancy with signs and symptoms listed previously or signs and symptoms of pregnancy-induced hypertension
   - Older adults
   - Patients with a history of alcoholism
   - Overweight patients
   - Malnourished patients
   - Patients on long-term drug therapies, such as steroids or hormonal therapy

Oral Glucose

Generic name	oral glucose
Trade name	Glutose, Insta-glucose
Mechanism of action	Increases the amount of sugar available for use as energy by the body
Indications	Patients with altered mental status who have a known history of diabetes controlled by medication and can swallow
Dosage	1 tube
Side effects	• None when given properly • May be aspirated by the patient without a gag reflex
Contraindications	• No permission by medical direction • Unresponsive • Unable to swallow • Known allergy to the glucose preparation

Seizures

- A seizure is a temporary change in behavior or consciousness caused by abnormal electrical activity within 1 or more groups of brain cells.

A seizure is a symptom of an underlying problem within the CNS.

- The most common cause of adult seizures in patients with a known seizure history is the failure to take anti-seizure medication. The most common cause of seizures in infants and young children is a high fever.

- Epilepsy is a condition of recurring seizures; the cause is usually irreversible.

- The type of seizure that involves stiffening and jerking of the patient's body is called a *tonic-clonic seizure* (formerly called a *grand mal seizure*). This type of seizure typically has 4 phases:
  1. Aura: a peculiar sensation that comes before a seizure.
  2. Tonic phase: The body's muscles stiffen, the patient's breathing may be noisy, and the patient may turn blue.
  3. Clonic phase: Alternating jerking and relaxation of the body occurs.
  4. Postictal phase: the period of recovery that follows a seizure, during which the patient often appears limp, has shallow breathing, and has an altered mental status.

- Status epilepticus is recurring seizures without an intervening period of consciousness. Status epilepticus is a medical emergency. It can cause brain damage or death if it is not treated.

Stroke

- A stroke is caused by the blockage or rupture of an artery supplying the brain. There are 2 main forms of stroke: ischemic and hemorrhagic.

    —Ischemic strokes are caused by a blood clot that decreases blood flow to the brain. Ischemic strokes can be further classified as either thrombotic or embolic.

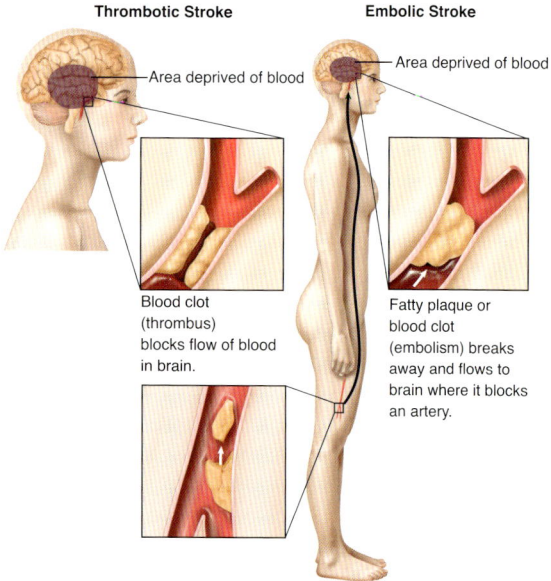

Thrombotic Stroke

Area deprived of blood

Blood clot (thrombus) blocks flow of blood in brain.

Embolic Stroke

Area deprived of blood

Fatty plaque or blood clot (embolism) breaks away and flows to brain where it blocks an artery.

- In a thrombotic stroke, a blood clot (thrombus) forms in a blood vessel of, or leading to, the brain.
- In an embolic stroke, a blood clot breaks up and travels through the circulatory system.
  —Hemorrhagic strokes (also called *cerebral hemorrhage*) are caused by bleeding into the brain.

Hemorrhagic Strokes

Subarachnoid hemorrhage

Intracerebral hemorrhage

Arachnoid

Area of bleeding

Ruptured aneurysm

Area of bleeding

Ruptured blood vessel

- Subarachnoid hemorrhage is caused by a ruptured blood vessel in the subarachnoid space, usually as a result of an aneurysm (an abnormal bulging of a blood vessel).
- Intracerebral hemorrhage is caused by a ruptured blood vessel within the brain itself (usually as a result of chronic high blood pressure).

- A transient ischemic attack (TIA) is a temporary interruption of the blood supply to the brain. Signs and symptoms completely resolve within 24 hours with no permanent damage.
- The Cincinnati Prehospital Stroke Scale is a useful tool that can be used to find out if a person who has an altered mental status might be having a stroke.

   —The Scale assesses 3 main areas:

   - Ask the patient to smile. Both sides of the face should move equally.
   - Ask the patient to close his eyes and raise his arms out in front of him. Both arms should move the same, or both arms should not move at all.
   - Ask the patient to say a simple sentence. The patient should be able to say the right words without slurring or forgetting or substituting words.

   —If the patient's response is not normal, request ALS personnel right away or begin transport to the closest appropriate facility.

Allergic Reactions

Signs and Symptoms by Body System

Body System	Signs and Symptoms
Respiratory	Tightness in the throat ("lump in the throat") or chest
	Coughing, rapid breathing, labored breathing, noisy breathing
	Hoarseness, stridor, difficulty talking, wheezing
Cardiovascular	Lightheadedness, fainting, weakness
	Increased heart rate, irregular heart rhythm
	Decreased blood pressure, circulatory collapse
Nervous	Restlessness, fear, panic, or a feeling of impending doom
	Headache
	Altered mental status to unresponsiveness
	Seizures

Skin (integumentary)	Warm, tingling feeling in the face, mouth, chest, feet, and hands
	Itching (pruritus), rash, hives (urticaria)
	Red skin (flushing); swelling of the face, neck, hands, feet and/or tongue
Gastrointestinal	Nausea, vomiting, abdominal cramps, pain
	Urgency to urinate, diarrhea
Generalized findings	Itchy, watery eyes; runny nose

Epinephrine

Generic name	epinephrine
Trade name	Adrenalin
Mechanism of action	Epinephrine works by relaxing the bronchial passages of the airway and constricting the blood vessels. The opening of the airway allows the patient to move more air into and out of the lungs, which will increase the amount of oxygen in the bloodstream. Constriction of the blood vessels slows the leakage of fluid from the blood vessels into the space around the cells of the body.

Indications	An EMT can assist a patient in using an epinephrine auto-injector if *all* of the following criteria are met: • The patient shows signs and symptoms of a severe allergic reaction, including respiratory distress and/or signs and symptoms of shock. • The patient has a physician-prescribed epinephrine auto-injector or the EMT's EMS system authorizes EMTs to carry the medication. • The EMT has specific authorization by medical direction.
Dosage	Adult: 1 adult auto-injector (0.3 mg) Infant and child: 1 infant/child auto-injector (0.15 mg)
Side effects	Rapid heart rate, anxiety, excitability, nausea, vomiting, chest pain or discomfort, headache, dizziness
Contraindications	There are no contraindications when used in a life-threatening situation.

Poisoning and Overdose

What Is a Poison?

- A poison is any substance taken into the body that interferes with normal body function.
- Poisoning is exposure to a substance that is harmful in any dosage.
- A toxin is a poisonous substance.
- An antidote is a substance that neutralizes a poison.
- A Poison Control Center is a medical facility that provides free telephone advice to the public and medical professionals in case of exposure to poisonous substances. In the United States, the national telephone number is 1-800-222-1222 (toll-free). This number is staffed 24 hours a day, 7 days a week, 365 days a year by pharmacists, physicians, nurses, and poison information providers.

Routes of Entry

- Toxins enter the body in 4 ways: ingestion, inhalation, injection, or absorption.

Examples of Common Poisons

Form of Poison	Examples
Solid	Medicines, plants, granulated detergent, granular pesticides, fertilizers, pool chemicals, disc batteries, chalk, clay, fabric softener, diaper pail deodorizer, toilet bowl deodorizer
Liquid	Syrup medicines, laundry soap, fabric softener, laundry bluing/brightening products, baby oil, bath oil/bubble bath, cream or lotion makeup, mouthwash, permanent wave solutions, hair removal products, rubbing alcohol, nail polish remover, furniture polish, lighter fluid, typewriter correction fluid, gasoline, kerosene, drain opener, disinfectants, toilet bowl cleaner, rust remover, pool chemicals, lamp oil, paint, antifreeze, windshield solution, brake fluid
Spray	Oven cleaner, glass cleaner, air freshener, insecticides, weed killer, spray paint, fabric softener, disinfectants

Gas	Carbon monoxide, automobile exhaust fumes, fumes from gas- or oil-burning stoves, tear gas, chlorine gas and pool chemicals, chemicals that workers are exposed to at industrial plants

Common Toxidromes

Toxidrome	Signs and Symptoms	Examples
Sympatho-mimetic (produces signs and symptoms like those of the sympathetic division of the autonomic nervous system)	Agitation, rapid breathing, increased heart rate, increased blood pressure, fever, seizures, sweating	Amphetamines, methamphetamines Cocaine Phencyclidine (PCP) Ecstasy Caffeine, pseudoephedrine (found in over-the-counter cold remedies)
Cholinergic	Altered mental status, decreased or increased	Organophosphate and carbamate insecticides

	heart rate, fever, seizures "SLUDGEM": • **S**alivation • **L**acrimation (tearing) • **U**rination • **D**efecation • **G**astro-intestinal distress • **E**mesls (vomiting) • **M**iosis (pupil constriction)	(ant sprays, flea sprays, and insect sprays, powders, and liquids) Some mushrooms Nerve agents (Sarin gas)
Anticho-linergic	Confusion, hallucinations, agitation, coma, blurred vision; warm, flushed, dry skin; dilated pupils	Antihistamines such as diphenhydramine (Benadryl) Jimson weed Tricyclic antidepressants such as amitriptyline (Elavil), desipramine (Norpramin), nortriptyline (Aventyl, Pamelor)

Opioid (narcotics)	Altered mental status, coma, slow or absent breathing, slow heart rate, low blood pressure, constricted pupils *Note:* Meperidine, propoxyphene, and diphenoxylate may cause dilated pupils.	Morphine Codeine Heroin Diphenoxylate (Lomotil) Meperidine (Demerol) Methadone (Dolophine) Propoxyphene (Darvon)
Sedative/ hypnotic (substances used to aid sleep, reduce anxiety, and treat depression, epilepsy, and high blood pressure)	Slurred speech, hallucinations, confusion, coma, respiratory depression, low blood pressure, pupil dilation or constriction, blurred vision, dry mouth, decreased temperature, staggering walk	Barbiturates (phenobarbital) Benzodiazepines [diazepam (Valium)] Alcohol GHB (a date rape drug, also called *liquid X*)

Activated Charcoal

Generic name	activated charcoal
Trade name	Liqui-Char, Actidose, InstaChar, SuperChar, and others
Mechanism of action	Activated charcoal acts as an adsorbent and will bind with many (but not all chemicals) and slow down or block absorption of the chemical by the body.
Indications	Poisoning by mouth
Dosage	Adults and children: 1 gram activated charcoal/kilogram of body weight
	Usual adult dose: 25 to 50 g
	Usual infant/child dose: 12.5 to 25 g
Side effects	Nausea, vomiting, abdominal cramping, constipation, black stools
Contraindications	• No permission by medical direction
	• Altered mental status
	• Inability to swallow
	• Ingestion of acids or alkalis

Environmental Emergencies

Mechanisms of Heat Loss

The body loses heat to the environment in 5 ways:

- Radiation is the transfer of heat from the surface of one object to the surface of another without contact between the 2 objects. When the temperature of the body is more than the temperature of the surroundings, the body will lose heat.
- Convection is the transfer of heat by the movement of air current. Wind speed affects heat loss by convection (wind-chill factor).
- Conduction is the transfer of heat between objects that are in direct contact. Heat flows from warmer areas to cooler ones.
- Evaporation is a loss of heat by vaporization of moisture on the body surface. The body will lose heat by evaporation if the skin temperature is higher than the temperature of the surroundings.
- The body loses heat through breathing. With normal breathing, the body continuously loses a relatively small amount of heat through the evaporation of moisture.

Hypothermia

- Hypothermia is a core body temperature of less than 95°F (35°C). This condition results when the body loses more heat than it gains or produces.
- Your main concern in providing care should be to remove the patient from the environment. Use trained rescuers for this purpose when necessary.

Assess the patient, keeping in mind that you need to move the patient to a warm location as quickly and as safely as possible. Remove any cold or wet clothing. Protect the patient from the environment. Assess the patient's mental status, airway, breathing, and circulation. Keep in mind that mental status decreases as the patient's body temperature drops.

- You may need to rewarm the patient. The 2 main types of rewarming are passive and active.

  —Passive rewarming is the warming of a patient with minimal or no use of heat sources other than the patient's own heat production. Passive rewarming methods include placing the patient in a warm environment, applying warm clothing and blankets, and preventing drafts.

  —Active rewarming should only be used if sustained warmth can be ensured. Active rewarming involves adding heat directly to the surface of the patient's body. Warm blankets, heat packs, and/or hot water bottles may be used, depending on how severe the hypothermia is.

Local Cold Injury

- Local cold injury (frostbite) involves tissue damage to a specific area of the body. It occurs when a body part, such as the nose, ears, cheeks, chin, hands, or feet, is exposed to prolonged or intense cold.

- A local cold injury may be early (superficial frostbite) or late (deep frostbite).

Superficial Cold Injury

- Skin first appears red and inflamed and becomes gray or white with continued cooling.
- Skin beneath the affected area remains soft.

Deep Cold Injury

- Whitish skin color is followed by a waxy appearance.
- Affected area becomes frozen; it feels stiff and solid.
- Patient may complain of a slight burning pain followed by a feeling of warmth and then numbness.
- Swelling and/or blisters may be present.
- If the affected area has thawed or partially thawed, skin may appear flushed, with areas that are blue, purple, pale, or mottled.

Hyperthermia

- When the body gains or produces more heat than it loses, hyperthermia (a high core body temperature) results.
- The 3 main types of heat emergencies are heat cramps, heat exhaustion, and heat stroke.
  - Heat cramps usually affect people who sweat a lot during strenuous activity in a warm environment. Water and electrolytes are lost from the body during sweating. This loss leads to dehydration and causes painful muscle spasms.

—Heat exhaustion is also a result of too much heat and dehydration. A patient with heat exhaustion usually sweats heavily. His body temperature is usually normal or slightly elevated. Severe heat exhaustion often requires intravenous fluids. Heat exhaustion may progress to heat stroke if it is not treated.

—Heat stroke is the most severe form of heat-related illness. It occurs when the body can no longer regulate its temperature. Most patients have hot, flushed skin and do not sweat. Individuals who wear heavy uniforms and perform strenuous activity for long periods in a hot environment are at risk for heat stroke.

- The first step in the emergency care of a patient suffering from a heat-related illness is to remove him from the hot environment. Move the patient to a cool (air-conditioned) location and follow treatment guidelines based on the patient's degree of heat-related illness.

Drowning

- Drowning is a process that results in harm to the respiratory system from submersion/immersion in a liquid.

- Delayed drowning (also called *secondary drowning*) occurs when a victim appears to have survived an immersion/submersion episode but later dies from respiratory failure or an infection.

- Immersion refers to covering of the face and airway in water or other fluid.

- In a submersion incident, the victim's entire body, including his airway, is under the water or other fluid.
- When providing emergency care for a drowning victim, ensure the safety of the rescue personnel.
- Suspect a possible spine injury if a diving accident is involved or unknown.
- Any breathless, pulseless patient who has been submerged in cold water should be resuscitated.

Special Considerations

Suspect neck injury:

- When the MOI is unknown
- When signs of facial trauma are present
- When signs of drug or alcohol use are present
- In incidents involving use of a water slide and in swimming, boating, water-skiing, or diving accidents

Bites and Stings

- Signs and symptoms of bites and stings typically include a history of a bite (spider, snake) or sting (insect, scorpion, marine animal), pain, redness, swelling, weakness, dizziness, chills, fever, nausea, and vomiting. Bite marks may be present.
- If a stinger is present, remove it by scraping the stinger out with the edge of card. Avoid using tweezers or forceps as these can squeeze venom from the venom sac into the wound.
- When caring for a victim of a bite or sting, watch closely for development of signs and symptoms of an allergic reaction; treat as needed.

Behavioral Emergencies

Behavior and Behavioral Change

- Behavior is the way in which a person acts or performs. It includes any or all of a person's activities, including physical and mental activity.
- Abnormal behavior is a way of acting or conducting one's self that:
  - —Is not consistent with society's norms and expectations
  - —Interferes with the individual's well-being and ability to function
  - —May be harmful to the individual or others
- A behavioral emergency is a situation in which a patient displays abnormal behavior that is unacceptable to the patient, family members, or community.

Factors That May Cause Changes in Behavior

Mind-Altering Substances	• Alcohol, drugs	
Situational Stressors	• Rape • Loss of a job • Career change • Death of a loved one • Marital stress or divorce	• Physical or psychological abuse • Natural disasters (tornado, flood, earthquake, hurricane)

Situational Stressors —cont'd		• Man-made disasters (war, explosion)
Medical Illnesses	• Poisoning • CNS infection • Head trauma • Seizure disorder • Lack of oxygen (hypoxia)	• Low blood sugar • Inadequate blood flow to the brain • Extremes of temperature (excessive cold or heat)
Psychiatric Illnesses or Crises	• Panic • Agitation • Bizarre thinking and behavior	• Self-destructive behavior, suicidal gesture (danger to self) • Threatening behavior, violence (danger to others)

Panic Attacks: Common Signs and Symptoms

- Numbness or tingling sensations (usually in the fingers, toes, or lips)
- Shortness of breath or a smothering sensation
- Heart palpitations (a rapid or irregular heartbeat)
- Fear of going crazy or being out of control
- Nausea or abdominal distress

- Choking
- Sweating
- Hot flashes or chills
- Feeling of detachment or being out of touch with one's self
- Trembling or shaking
- Dizziness or faintness
- Fear of becoming seriously ill or dying

Common Phobias

Specific Phobias	Social Phobias
- Animals (especially insects or spiders) - Thunder and/or lightning - Doctors or dentists - Germs, bacteria - Being alone - Blood, injection, or injury - Situations (heights, enclosed places, elevators, crossing bridges, driving or riding in vehicles, airplane travel)	- Public speaking - Eating in public - Using public restrooms - Writing while others are looking on - Performing publicly

Depression: Signs and Symptoms

- Loss of appetite
- Diarrhea or constipation
- Tiredness
- Difficulty sleeping or sleeping too much
- Muscle aches
- Vague pains
- Significant weight loss or gain
- A loss of interest in usual activities or hobbies
- Crying spells
- An inability to make decisions or concentrate
- Constant feelings of sadness, irritability, or tension
- Feelings of anger, helplessness, guilt, worthlessness, hopelessness, or loneliness
- Thoughts of suicide or death

Suicide: Risk Factors

- Previous suicide attempt(s)
- History of mental disorders, particularly depression
- History of alcohol and/or substance abuse
- Family history of suicide
- Family history of child maltreatment
- Easy access to lethal methods
- Unwillingness to seek help because of the stigma attached to mental health and substance abuse disorders or suicidal thoughts

- Feelings of hopelessness
- Impulsive or aggressive tendencies
- Barriers to accessing mental health treatment
- Loss (relational, social, work, or financial)
- Physical illness
- Cultural and religious beliefs; for example, the belief that suicide is a noble resolution of a personal problem
- Local epidemics of suicide
- Isolation, a feeling of being cut off from other people

Calming Patients with Behavioral Emergencies

- Acknowledge that the person seems upset, and restate that you are there to help.
- Inform the person of what you are doing.
- Ask questions in a calm, reassuring voice.
- Maintain a comfortable distance.
- Encourage the patient to state what is troubling him.
- Do not make quick moves.
- Respond honestly to patient's questions.
- Do not threaten, challenge, or argue with a disturbed patient.
- Tell the truth; do not lie to the patient.
- Do not "play along" with the patient's visual or auditory disturbances.
- Involve trusted family members or friends.

- Be prepared to stay at scene for a long time. Always remain with the patient.
- Avoid unnecessary physical contact. Call for additional help if needed.
- Use good eye contact.

Documenting the Use of Restraints

When caring for a patient in restraints, document the following information:

- The reason for the restraints
- The number of personnel used to restrain the patient
- The type of restraint used
- The time the restraints were placed on the patient
- The status of the patient's ABCs and distal pulses before and after the restraints were applied
- Reassessment of the patient's ABCs and distal pulses

Obstetrics and Gynecology
Vaginal Bleeding in Late Pregnancy

Signs and Symptoms	Placenta Previa	Abruptio Placenta	Uterine Rupture
Vaginal bleeding	Sudden Bright red	May be absent (concealed or hidden) If seen, may be moderate to severe; usually dark red	May or may not be present
Abdominal pain	Usually none (**P**ainless = **P**revia)	Sudden, severe	Sudden, severe Abdomen tender, rigid Possible contractions
Signs of shock	Likely	Yes; may seem out of proportion to amount of blood loss seen	Yes

Fetal movement	Usually present	Decreased	Absent
		May be absent	

Stages of Labor

Stage 1: Begins with the onset of uterine contractions; ends with a complete thinning out and opening of the cervix

Stage 2: Begins with opening of the cervix; ends with delivery of the infant

Stage 3: Begins with delivery of the infant; ends with delivery of the placenta

True Labor and False Labor Contractions

True Labor Contractions	False Labor Contractions
Occur regularly	Usually weak, irregular
Get closer together	Do not get closer together over time
Become stronger as time passes; each lasts about 30 to 60 seconds	Do not get stronger
Continue despite patient's activity	May stop or slow down when the patient walks, lies down, or changes position

Signs of Imminent Delivery

Consider delivering at the scene when

- Delivery can be expected in a few minutes.
- Crowning is present.
- Contractions are regular, lasting 45 to 60 seconds, and are 1 to 2 minutes apart.
- No suitable transportation is available.
- The hospital cannot be reached because of heavy traffic, bad weather, a natural disaster, or a similar situation.

Apgar Score

Sign	0	1	2
Appearance (color)	Blue or pale	Body pink Extremities blue	Completely pink
Pulse (heart rate)	Absent	< 100/min	> 100/min
Grimace (irritability)	No response	Grimace	Cough, sneeze, cry
Activity (muscle tone)	Limp	Some flexion of extremities	Active motion
Respirations (respiratory effort)	Absent	Slow, irregular	Good, crying

Bleeding and Shock

External Bleeding

Types of Bleeding

	Arterial	Venous	Capillary
Color	Bright red	Dark red, maroon	Dark red
Blood Flow	Spurts with each heartbeat	Flows steadily	Oozes slowly
Bleeding Control	Difficult to control	Usually easier to control than arterial bleeding; bleeding from deep veins may be hard to control	Often clots and stops by itself within a few minutes

Measures of Severe Blood Loss

Patient Type	Normal Blood Volume	Severe Blood Loss
Adult	5000-6000 mL	Loss of ≥1000 mL

Child (8-year-old)	2000 mL	Loss of ≥500 mL
Infant	800 mL	Loss of ≥100-200 mL

Internal Bleeding

Possible Signs and Symptoms of Internal Bleeding

Signs and symptoms of internal bleeding may develop quickly or may take hours or days to develop. Signs and symptoms include:

- Pain, tenderness, swelling, or discoloration of the skin (bruising) in the injured area
- A weak, rapid pulse
- Pale, cool, moist skin
- Broken ribs or bruising on the chest
- Vomiting or coughing up bright red blood or dark, "coffee-ground" blood
- A tender, rigid, and/or swollen abdomen
- Bleeding from the mouth, rectum, vagina, or another body opening
- Black (tarry) stools or stools with bright red blood

Shock

Causes of Shock

Shock can be caused by failure of the body's pump (the heart), fluid (blood), or container (the blood vessels).

- Pump failure
  - —The amount of blood the heart pumps throughout the body depends on how many times the heart beats and the force of the contractions.
  - —Cardiogenic shock can result if the heart beats too quickly or too slowly or if the heart muscle does not have enough force to pump blood effectively to all parts of the body.
  - —This type of shock can occur because of a heart attack, a heart rhythm that is too fast or too slow, an injury to the heart, or other conditions that affect the heart's ability to pump.
- Fluid loss
  - —Shock can result if there is not enough blood for the heart to pump through the cardiovascular system.
  - —Shock caused by severe bleeding is called *hemorrhagic shock.* The bleeding may be internal, external, or both.
  - —Shock caused by a loss of blood, plasma, or other body fluid is called *hypovolemic shock.*
- Container failure
  - —When shock caused by container failure occurs, the blood vessels lose their ability to adjust the flow of blood. Instead of expanding and constricting as needed, the blood vessels remain enlarged. The amount of fluid in the body remains constant (there is no actual loss of fluid), but blood pools in the outer areas of the body.
  - —The 4 major causes of this type of shock are:
    - Injury to the spinal cord (neurogenic shock)

- Severe infection (septic shock)
- Severe allergic reaction (anaphylactic shock)
- Severe drug reaction

Early Shock: Signs and Symptoms

Anxiety, restlessness

Thirst

Nausea/vomiting

Increased respiratory rate

Slight increase in heart rate

Pale, cool, moist skin

Blood pressure in normal range

Late Shock: Signs and Symptoms

Slow to respond, confused or unresponsive

If awake, extreme thirst

Nausea/vomiting

Shallow, labored, irregular breathing

Rapid heart rate

Cool, moist skin that is pale, blue, or mottled

Low blood pressure

115

Soft-Tissue Injuries

Compartment Syndrome: Possible Causes

- Compression injury
- Strenuous exercise
- Circumferential burns
- Frostbite
- Constrictive bandages, splints, casts
- Animal/insect bites
- Bleeding disorders
- Arterial bleeding
- Soft-tissue injury
- Fracture

The "Five Ps" of Compartment Syndrome

- *P*ain on passive stretching of the muscle
- *P*aralysis (or weakness)
- *P*aresthesias
- Increased *p*ressure
- Diminished *p*eripheral pulses

Crush Syndrome: Possible Mechanisms of Injury

- Mine cave-ins
- Trench collapse
- Motor vehicle crashes
- Landslide, avalanche, rockslide
- Rubble from war, earthquake

- Pinning under heavy objects (such as a tractor)
- Severe beatings

Open Chest Injuries

- Apply an airtight dressing and seal it on 3 sides.
- Place the patient in a position of comfort if no spinal injury is suspected.

Impaled Objects

- Do not remove the impaled object unless it is through the cheek or it interferes with airway management or chest compressions.
- Manually secure the object.
- Expose the wound area.
- Control bleeding.
- Use a bulky dressing to help stabilize the object.

Eviscerations

- Do not attempt to replace protruding organs.
- Cover with a thick, moist dressing.

Amputations

- Locate the amputated part.
- Put the amputated part in a dry plastic bag or waterproof container.
- Seal the bag or container and place it in water that contains a few ice cubes.
- Immobilize the injured area to prevent further injury.
- Treat the patient for shock and keep him warm.
- Transport the amputated part with the patient to an appropriate facility.

Open Neck Wounds

- Immediately place a gloved hand over the wound to control bleeding.
- Cover the wound with an airtight (occlusive) dressing.
- Apply a bulky dressing over the occlusive dressing. To control bleeding, apply pressure over the dressing with a gloved hand. Make sure not to press on the trachea, or you may cause an airway obstruction.
- Apply a pressure bandage. Wrap it across the injured side of the neck and under the opposite armpit. *Never apply a circular bandage around a patient's neck.* Strangulation can occur.
- Treat the patient for shock.

Burns

A superficial (first-degree) burn involves only the outer layer of the skin. Symptoms include:

- Reddening of the skin
- Swelling

A partial-thickness (second-degree) burn involves the outer and middle layers of the skin. Symptoms include:

- Deep, intense pain
- Reddening, blisters

A full-thickness (third-degree) burn extends through all layers of the skin. Symptoms include:

- Deep, intense pain
- Reddening, blisters
- Areas of charred skin

Rule of Nines

Body Area	Adult	Child	Infant
Head and neck	9%	18%	18%
Front of trunk	18%	18%	18%
Back of trunk	18%	18%	18%
Each arm (shoulder to fingertips)	9%	9%	9%
Each leg (groin to toe)	18%	13.5%	13.5%
Genitals	1%	1%	1%

Musculoskeletal Care

Musculoskeletal Injuries: Signs and Symptoms

- Pain or tenderness over the injury site
- Swelling
- Deformity, angulation (abnormal position of an extremity)
- Crepitation (grating sensation or sound)
- Limited movement
- Joint locked into position
- Exposed bone ends
- Bruising
- Bleeding
- One extremity appears to be a different length, shape, or size than the other
- Loss of pulse or sensation below the injury site

Reasons for Splinting

- To limit the motion of bone fragments, bone ends, or dislocated joints
- To lessen the damage to muscles, nerves, or blood vessels caused by broken bones
- To help prevent a closed injury from becoming an open injury
- To lessen the restriction of blood flow caused by bone ends or dislocations compressing blood vessels
- To reduce bleeding resulting from tissue damage caused by bone ends

- To reduce pain associated with the movement of the bone and the joint
- To reduce the risk of paralysis due to a damaged spine

Hazards of Improper Splinting

- The compression of nerves, tissues, and blood vessels from the splint
- A delay in transport of a patient with a life-threatening injury
- Distal circulation that is reduced because of the splint's being applied too tightly to the extremity
- Aggravating the musculoskeletal injury
- Causing or aggravating tissue, nerve, vessel, or muscle damage from excessive bone or joint movement

General Rules of Splinting

Follow these general guidelines when splinting a musculoskeletal injury:

- Take BSI precautions and wear appropriate personal protective equipment (PPE). In most situations, the patient should not be moved before splinting unless he is in danger.
- If possible, remove or cut away clothing to expose the injury. Remove jewelry from the injured area.

- Assess pulses, movement, and sensation distal to the injury before and after applying a splint. You may find it helpful to lightly mark the pulse location with a pen to save time when rechecking pulses. Assess pulses, movement, and sensation every 15 minutes and document your findings.
- Cover open wounds with a sterile dressing.
- Before applying a rigid or semi-rigid splint, pad it to reduce patient discomfort caused by pressure, especially around bony areas.
- Splint the area above and below the injury. If a bone is injured, immobilize the joint above and below the injury. If a joint is injured, immobilize the bone above and below the injury.
- Before splinting an injured hand or foot, place it in the position of function. Do not place the hand or foot in a position of function if you find it in an abnormal position and meet resistance or cause pain when you attempt to place it in the position of function.
- Pad the hollow areas (voids) between the splint and the extremity.
- Do not intentionally replace protruding bones. During the splinting process, bone ends may be drawn back into the wound. This is to be expected and is acceptable.
- Avoid excessive movement of the injured area when applying a splint.
- When securing the splint to the injured area, avoid placing ties or straps directly over the injury.

- Splint the injury before moving the patient unless he is in danger or life-threatening conditions exist.
- When in doubt about whether a musculoskeletal injury is present, splint the injury.
- If the patient shows signs of shock, align him in the anatomical position on a long backboard.

Warning Signs That a Splint Is Too Tight

- The patient's fingers or toes become cold to the touch in the splinted extremity.
- The patient's fingers or toes begin to turn pale or blue in the splinted extremity.
- The patient is unable to move fingers or toes in the splinted extremity.
- The patient experiences increased pain in the splinted extremity.
- The patient experiences increased swelling below the splint.
- The patient complains of numbness or tingling in the extremity.
- The patient complains of burning or stinging in the splinted extremity.

Injuries to the Head and Spine

Possible Spinal Injury: Signs and Symptoms

- Tenderness in the injured area
- Pain associated with movement (Do not ask the patient to move to see if he has pain. Do not move the patient to test for a pain response).
- Pain independent of movement
- Pain on palpation along the spinal column
- Pain down the lower legs or into the rib cage
- Pain that comes and goes, usually along the spine and/or the lower legs
- Soft-tissue injuries associated with trauma to the head and neck (cuts, bruises)
- Numbness, weakness, or tingling in the extremities
- A loss of sensation or paralysis below the site of injury
- A loss of sensation or paralysis in the upper or lower extremities
- Difficulty breathing
- A loss of bladder or bowel control
- An inability of the patient to walk, move his extremities, or feel sensation
- Deformity or muscle spasm along the spinal column

Rapid Extrication

Rapid extrication is an example of an urgent move.

Indications

- Unsafe scene
- Altered mental status
- Inadequate breathing
- Shock (hypoperfusion)
- Patient blocks access to another, more seriously injured patient

Helmet Removal

Do not assume that a helmet must be removed. If your patient has a spinal injury, removing the helmet could worsen the injury. To determine if a helmet should be left in place or removed, you should first ask yourself the following questions:

- Can I access the patient's airway?
- Is the patient's airway clear?
- Is the patient breathing adequately?
- Is there room to apply a face mask if it is necessary to assist the patient's breathing?
- How well does the helmet fit?
- Can the patient's head move within the helmet?
- Can the patient's spine be stabilized in a neutral position if the helmet is left in place?

You should leave a helmet in place in the following circumstances:

- There are no impending airway or breathing problems.
- The helmet fits well, with little or no movement of the patient's head within the helmet.

125

- Helmet removal would cause further injury to the patient.
- Proper spinal stabilization can be performed with the helmet in place.
- The presence of the helmet does not interfere with your ability to assess and reassess airway and breathing.

You should remove a helmet in these circumstances:

- You are unable to assess and/or reassess the patient's airway and breathing.
- The helmet limits your ability to adequately manage the patient's airway or breathing.
- The helmet does not fit properly, allowing excessive head movement within the helmet.
- You cannot properly stabilize the patient's spine with the helmet in place.
- The patient is in cardiac arrest.

Skull Fracture: Signs and Symptoms

- Bruises or cuts to the scalp
- Deformity to the skull
- Discoloration around the eyes (raccoon eyes)
- Discoloration behind the ears (Battle's sign)
- Loss of consciousness
- Confusion
- Convulsions
- Restlessness, irritability
- Drowsiness

- Blood or clear, watery fluid (cerebrospinal fluid) leaking from the ears or nose
- Visual disturbances
- Changes in pupils (unequal pupil size or pupils that are not reactive to light)
- Slurred speech
- Difficulties with balance
- Stiff neck
- Vomiting

Traumatic Head Injury: Signs and Symptoms

- Changes in mental status that range from confusion and repetitive questioning to unresponsiveness
- Deep cuts or tears to the scalp or face
- Exposed brain tissue (a very bad sign)
- Penetrating injuries such as from gunshot wounds and impaled objects
- Swelling ("goose eggs"), bruising of the skin
- Edges or fragments of bone seen or felt through the skin
- A deformity of the skull, such as "sunken" areas (depressions)
- Swelling or discoloration behind the ears (Battle's sign; may not be seen for hours after the injury)
- Swelling or discoloration around the eyes (raccoon eyes; may not be seen for hours after the injury)
- Pupils that are unequal in size or irregular in shape or that do not react to light equally; dilation of both pupils

- An irregular breathing pattern
- Nausea and/or vomiting
- Seizures
- Blood or clear, watery fluid from the ears or nose
- Weakness or numbness of one side of the body
- A deterioration in vital signs
- A loss of bladder or bowel control

Injuries to the Brain

- A concussion is a traumatic brain injury that results in a temporary loss of function in some or all of the brain. A concussion occurs when the head strikes an object or is struck by an object. The injury may or may not cause a loss of consciousness. A headache, loss of appetite, vomiting, and pale skin are common soon after the injury.

- A cerebral contusion is a brain injury in which brain tissue is bruised and damaged in a local area. Bruising may occur at both the area of direct impact (coup) and/or on the side opposite (contrecoup) the impact.

- A subdural hematoma usually results from tearing of veins located between the dura and the cerebral cortex after an injury to the head. Blood builds up in the space between the dura and the arachnoid layer of the meninges.

- An epidural hematoma involves a rapid buildup of blood between the dura and the skull. An epidural hematoma often involves the tearing of an artery, usually the middle meningeal artery.

- An intracerebral hematoma is a collection of blood within the brain. Signs and symptoms depend on the area of the brain involved, the amount of bleeding, and associated injuries.
- An altered or decreasing mental status is the best indicator of a brain injury.

Injuries to the Chest, Abdomen, and Genitalia

Deadly and Potentially Deadly Chest Injuries

Deadly Chest Injuries	Potentially Deadly Chest Injuries
Tension pneumothorax Open pneumothorax Massive hemothorax Cardiac tamponade Flail chest	Pulmonary contusion Myocardial contusion

Rib Fracture: Signs and Symptoms

- Localized pain at the fracture site that worsens with deep breathing, coughing, or moving
- Self-splinting of the injury by holding the arm close to the chest
- Pain on inspiration
- Shallow breathing
- Tenderness on palpation
- Deformity of the chest wall
- Crepitus
- Swelling and/or bruising at the fracture site
- Possible subcutaneous emphysema

Flail Chest: Signs and Symptoms

- Crepitus
- Breathing difficulty
- Bruising of the chest wall
- Increased heart rate (tachycardia)
- Pain and self-splinting of the affected side
- Increased respiratory rate (tachypnea)
- Pain in the chest associated with breathing
- Paradoxical chest wall movement

Simple Pneumothorax: Signs and Symptoms

- Sudden onset of sharp pain in the chest associated with breathing
- Shortness of breath
- Difficulty breathing
- Decreased or absent breath sounds on the affected side
- Increased respiratory rate (tachypnea)
- Increased heart rate (tachycardia)
- Subcutaneous emphysema (may not be present)

Tension Pneumothorax: Signs and Symptoms

- Cool, clammy skin
- Increased pulse rate
- Cyanosis (late sign)

- JVD
- Decreased blood pressure
- Severe respiratory distress
- Agitation, restlessness, anxiety
- Bulging of intercostal muscles on the affected side
- Decreased or absent breath sounds on the affected side
- Tracheal deviation toward the unaffected side (late sign)
- Possible subcutaneous emphysema in the face, neck, or chest wall

Hemothorax: Signs and Symptoms

- Cool, clammy skin
- Weak, thready pulse
- Restlessness, agitation, anxiety
- Coughing up blood (hemoptysis) (may not occur)
- Rapid, shallow breathing (tachypnea)
- Flat neck veins (resulting from hypovolemia)
- Decreasing blood pressure (hypotension)
- Decreased or absent breath sounds on the affected side

Cardiac Tamponade: Signs and Symptoms

- Cool, clammy skin
- Normal breath sounds
- Narrowing pulse pressure

- Trachea in midline position
- Increased heart rate (tachycardia)
- Cyanosis of head, neck, upper extremities
- Muffled heart sounds (often difficult to assess in the field)
- Distended neck veins (may not be present in hypovolemia)

Traumatic Asphyxia: Signs and Symptoms

- JVD
- Swelling of the tongue and lips
- Eyes that may appear bloodshot and bulging
- Deep red, purple, or blue discoloration of the head and neck ("hooding")
- Low blood pressure once the compression is released
- Skin that remains pink below the level of the crush injury (unless other injuries are present)

Pulmonary Contusion: Signs and Symptoms

- Signs of blunt chest trauma
- Restlessness, anxiety
- Increased respiratory rate
- Increased heart rate
- Cough
- Coughing up blood (hemoptysis)

- Chest pain
- Difficulty breathing
- Cyanosis

Open Pneumothorax: Signs and Symptoms

- Shortness of breath
- Increased heart rate
- Pain at the site of injury
- Increased respiratory rate
- Subcutaneous emphysema
- Sucking sound on inhalation
- Open wound in the chest wall
- Decreased breath sounds on the affected side

Abdominal Injury: Signs and Symptoms

- Patient lies still, usually on his side, with the legs drawn up to the chest (fetal position)
- Nausea
- Vomiting blood (hematemesis)
- Possible blood in the urine (hematuria)
- Possible skin wounds and penetrations
- Abdominal pain

- Rigid abdominal muscles
- Distended abdomen
- Rapid, shallow breathing
- Signs of shock
- Protruding organs (evisceration)

Infant and Child Emergency Care

Age Classifications of Infants and Children

Life Stage	Age
Newly born infant	Birth to several hours following birth
Neonate	Birth to 1 month
Infant	1 to 12 months of age • Young infant: 0 to 6 months of age • Older infant: 6 months to 1 year of age
Toddler	1 to 3 years of age
Preschooler	4 to 5 years of age
School-age child	6 to 12 years of age
Adolescent	13 to 18 years of age

Developmental Stages

Infants (Birth to 1 Year of Age)

- They are completely dependent on others.
- Young infants (0 to 6 months of age) are unafraid of strangers and have no modesty.
- Older infants (6 months to 1 year of age) do not like to be separated from their caregiver (separation anxiety). They may be threatened by direct eye contact with strangers. They show little modesty.
- Watch the baby from a distance before making contact.

- Assess the baby on the caregiver's lap if possible.
- Handle an infant gently but firmly, always supporting the head and neck if the baby is not on a solid surface.

Toddlers (1 to 3 Years of Age)

- Eye-hand coordination improves, and sitting, standing, and walking begin. As a result, toddlers are prone to injury.
- They respond appropriately to an angry or friendly voice.
- They have strong separation anxiety when separated from their primary caregiver.
- You cannot reason with a toddler.
- They are likely to be more cooperative if they are given a comfort object, like a blanket, stuffed animal, or toy.
- They are distrustful of strangers and are likely to resist examination and treatment.
- When possible, allow the child to remain on the caregiver's lap. If this is not possible, try to keep the caregiver within the child's line of vision.
- Replace clothing promptly after assessing each body area.

Preschoolers (4 to 5 Years of Age)

- They are afraid of the unknown, the dark, being left alone, and adults who look or act mean.

- They may think their illness or injury is punishment for bad behavior or thoughts. Assure the child that he was not bad and is not being punished.
- Use simple words and phrases and a reassuring tone of voice.
- They do not like being touched or having their clothing removed. Remove clothing, assess the child, and then quickly replace clothing.
- Allow the caregiver to remain with the child whenever possible.
- Encourage the child's participation. Tell the child how things will feel and what is to be done just before doing it.

School-Age Children (6 to 12 Years of Age)

- They are usually cooperative.
- They fear pain, permanent injury, disfigurement, blood, and prolonged separation from their caregiver.
- They are very modest and do not like their bodies exposed to strangers.
- They may view illness or injury as punishment. Reassure them that how they feel or what is happening is not related to being punished.
- Talk directly to the child about what happened, even if you also obtain a history from the caregiver.
- Explain procedures before carrying them out. Be honest.
- Allow the child to see and touch equipment that may be used in his care.

Adolescents (13 to 18 Years of Age)

- They often show inconsistent and unpredictable behavior.
- If possible, obtain a history from the patient instead of a caregiver.
- Explain things clearly and honestly. Allow time for questions.
- Allow the caregiver to be present during your assessment, if the patient wishes. However, some adolescents may prefer to be assessed privately, away from their caregiver.
- When caring for an adolescent, do not tease or embarrass him, particularly in front of his peers.

Vital Signs

Normal Respiratory Rates in Children at Rest

Life Stage	Age	Breaths per Minute
Newborn	Birth to 1 month	30-50
Infant	1 to 12 months	20-40
Toddler	1 to 3 years	20-30
Preschooler	4 to 5 years	20-30
School-age child	6 to 12 years	16-30
Adolescent	13 to 18 years	12-20

Normal Heart Rates in Children at Rest

Life Stage	Age	Beats per Minute
Newborn	Birth to 1 month	120-160
Infant	1 to 12 months	80-140
Toddler	1 to 3 years	80-130
Preschooler	4 to 5 years	80-120
School-age child	6 to 12 years	70-110
Adolescent	13 to 18 years	60-100

Lower Limit of Normal Systolic Blood Pressure by Age

Life Stage	Age	Lower Limit of Normal Systolic Blood Pressure
Term neonate	0 to 28 days	>60 mm Hg or strong central pulse
Infant	1 to 12 months	>70 mm Hg or strong central pulse
Child/Adolescent	1 to 10 years	>70 + (2 × age in years)
	≥10 years	>90 mm Hg

Common Problems in Infants and Children

Signs of Respiratory Distress

- Alertness, irritability, anxiousness, restlessness
- Noisy breathing (stridor, grunting, gurgling, wheezing)
- A breathing rate that is faster than normal for the patient's age
- An increased depth of breathing
- Nasal flaring
- A mild increase in the heart rate
- Retractions
- Head bobbing
- Seesaw respirations (abdominal breathing)
- The use of neck muscles to breathe
- Changes in skin color

Signs of Respiratory Failure

- Sleepiness or agitation
- Combativeness
- Limpness; may be unable to sit up without help
- A breathing rate that is initially fast with periods of slowing and then eventually slowing
- An altered mental status
- A shallow chest rise
- Nasal flaring

- Retractions
- Head bobbing
- Pale, mottled, or bluish skin
- Weak peripheral pulses

Cardiopulmonary Failure: Signs and Symptoms

- Mental status changes
- Weak respiratory effort
- Slow, shallow breathing
- Pale, mottled, or bluish skin
- A slow pulse rate
- Weak central pulses and absent peripheral pulses
- Cool extremities
- A delayed capillary refill

Altered Mental Status: Possible Causes

- A low blood oxygen level (hypoxia)
- Head trauma
- Seizures
- Brain infection
- Shock
- Low blood sugar
- Drug or alcohol ingestion
- Fever
- Respiratory failure

Shock: Possible Causes

- Shock rarely results from a primary cardiac problem in infants and children.
- Common causes of shock in infants and children include diarrhea and dehydration, trauma, vomiting, blood loss, infection, and abdominal injuries.
- Less common causes of shock include allergic reactions, poisoning, and cardiac disorders.

Seizures: Possible Causes

- A low blood oxygen level
- Low blood sugar
- Brain tumor
- Poisoning
- Head injury
- Previous brain damage
- Seizure disorder
- Fever
- Infection
- An abnormal heart rhythm
- Inherited factors
- Unknown cause

Sudden Infant Death Syndrome

- The National Institute of Child Health and Human Development defines sudden infant death syndrome (SIDS) as "the sudden and unexpected death of an infant that remains unexplained after a thorough case investigation, including performance of a complete autopsy, examination of the death scene, and review of the clinical history."

- About 90% of all SIDS deaths occur during the first 6 months of life. Most deaths occur between the ages of 2 and 4 months.

- SIDS occurs in apparently healthy infants. Boys are affected more often than girls. Most SIDS deaths occur at home, usually during the night after a period of sleep. The baby is most often discovered in the early morning.

- The cause of SIDS is not clearly understood. Research is ongoing.

- Common SIDS physical exam findings include an unresponsive baby who is not breathing and has no pulse. The skin often appears blue or mottled. You may see frothy sputum or vomitus around the mouth and nose. The underside of the baby's body may look dark and bruised because of pooled blood (dependent lividity). General stiffening of the body (rigor mortis) may be present.

- An apparent life-threatening event (ALTE) is also called *near-miss SIDS* or *near-SIDS.*
  - —An ALTE is an episode in which an infant was about to die but was found early enough for successful resuscitation.
  - —The infant has some combination of apnea (absence of breathing), color change (cyanosis or pallor), marked change in muscle tone (usually extreme limpness), and choking or gagging.
- Try to resuscitate unless signs of obvious death are present.
- Caregivers will be in agony from emotional distress, remorse, and guilt. Avoid any comments that might suggest blame to the caregiver.

Trauma

- Injuries are the leading cause of death in infants and children.
- Blunt trauma is the most common mechanism of serious injury in the pediatric patient.

- Causes of common blunt trauma injuries include
  —Falls
  —Bicycle-related injuries
  —Motor vehicle–related injuries (restrained and unrestrained passengers)
  —Car-pedestrian incidents
  —Drowning, near drowning
  —Sports-related injuries
  —Abuse and neglect

Child Abuse and Neglect

- Child maltreatment: An act or failure to act by a parent, a caregiver, or another person as defined by state law that results in physical abuse, neglect, medical neglect, sexual abuse, emotional abuse, or an act or failure to act that presents an impending risk of serious harm to a child
- Physical abuse: Physical acts that caused or could have caused physical injury to the child
- Neglect: Failure to provide for a child's basic needs; can be medical, physical, educational, or emotional

Signs of neglect that you may see in the child's environment include:

- Untreated chronic illness (such as a diabetic or an asthmatic child with no medication)
- Untreated soft-tissue injuries
- A home that is bug- or rodent-infested

- A lack of adult supervision
- A lack of food or basic necessities
- A child who appears to be malnourished
- Stool or urine present on items in the home
- An unsafe living environment
- The presence of drugs or alcohol paraphernalia

Physical signs that may indicate abuse include:

- Multiple bruises in various stages of healing
- Human bite marks
- Inflicted burns: "stocking-like" burns with no associated splash marks, usually present on the buttocks, genitalia, or extremities
- Circular burns from a cigarette or cigar
- Rope burns on the wrists
- Burns in the shape of a household utensil or appliance, such as a spoon or an iron
- Fractures
- Head, face, and oral injuries
- Abdominal injuries
- An injury inconsistent with the history or developmental level of the child

Emergency Care of Abused and Neglected Children

- Reporting of known or suspected child abuse is required by law in most states.

- Do not accuse the caregiver in the field.

- Remain objective. Report what you see and what you hear. Do not comment on what you think.

Emergency Vehicle Operations

When to Notify Dispatch

- Receiving the call
- Responding to the call
- Arriving at the scene
- Leaving the scene for the receiving facility
- Arriving at the receiving facility
- Leaving the hospital for the station
- Arriving at the station

Response Action List

- Verify the location and type of call.
- Select the most appropriate route.
- Observe weather and road conditions, and modify response if needed.
- Apply safety restraint devices.
- Notify dispatch agency of your response.
- Modify your emergency response on the basis of knowledge of the characteristics of your response vehicle. Factors such as length, width, and weight will alter the way your vehicle handles.
- Understand appropriate use of lights and siren.
- Obtain additional information from dispatch.
- Drive with due regard for the safety of others.
- Maintain a safe following distance.
- Approach the scene from uphill and upwind as needed.

Contributing Factors to Unsafe Driving Conditions

- Escorts
- Road surface
- Excessive speed
- Reckless driving
- Weather conditions
- Multiple-vehicle response
- Inadequate dispatch information and unfamiliarity with the location
- Failing to heed traffic warning signals
- Disregarding traffic rules and regulations
- Failing to anticipate the actions of other motorists
- Failing to obey traffic signals or posted speed limits

Air Medical Transport Considerations

MOI that may require helicopter transport include:

- A vehicle rollover with unrestrained passengers
- An incident in which a vehicle strikes a pedestrian at a speed greater than 10 miles per hour
- Falls from a height greater than 15 feet
- An incident in which a motorcyclist is thrown from the motorcycle at a speed of more than 20 miles per hour
- Multiple victims
- Time and distance must also be considered before transporting by helicopter. Helicopter transport should be considered when

—The transport time to a trauma center is more than 15 minutes by ground ambulance.

—The transport time to a local hospital by ground ambulance is more than the transport time to a trauma center by helicopter.

—The patient is entrapped and extrication will take longer than 15 minutes.

—Using local ground ambulance leaves the local community without ground ambulance coverage.

—The patient needs rapid transport to a specialty center (e.g., a burn center or pediatric center).

Helicopter Safety

- Never move toward a helicopter until signaled by the flight crew.

- Always approach from the front so that the pilot can see you.

- Wear ear and eye protection when approaching the helicopter.

- Never raise your arms or equipment above your head.

- Remove loose items, such as hats, that can be blown around or sucked into the rotors or engines.

- If the aircraft is parked on a slope, always approach and exit from the downhill side.

- When moving from one side of the helicopter to the other, always cross in front of the helicopter.

- Do not open or pull on any part of the aircraft.

- Do not allow vehicles or non-aircraft personnel within 60 feet of the aircraft.

Gaining Access

Hazard Control and Safety Considerations

Be alert for any of the following:

- Traffic at the scene
- Gasoline spills
- Hazardous materials
- Exposed or downed electrical wires
- Fire or the possibility of fire
- Explosive materials
- An unstable vehicle or structure
- Environmental conditions (heavy rain, heavy snow fall, flash floods)

Extrication

- Simple extrication is the use of hand tools in order to gain access and extricate the patient from the vehicle. Simple hand tools include hammers, hacksaws, battery-operated saws, and pry bars.
- Complex extrication involves the use of powered hydraulic rescue tools such as cutters, spreaders, and rams.
- The patient's level of entrapment will determine whether the extrication will fall into a simple or complex category.

Degrees of Entrapment

- No entrapment
- Light entrapment
  - —In most cases, only hand tools are needed to gain access to the patient.
- Moderate entrapment
  - —Usually hydraulic, gas, or electric tools are required to remove the doors from the vehicle.
  - —The same tools can remove the roof and any additional pieces of the vehicle that need to be removed in order to gain patient access and provide egress.
- Heavy entrapment
  - —Rescuers are required to actually move a structural component of the vehicle to free the patient for removal from the vehicle.

Special Response Situations

Levels of Personal Protective Equipment

Level	When Used	Notes
A	Intended for situations where chemical(s) have been identified and pose high levels of hazards to the respiratory system, skin, and eyes	• Vapor protective suit that is encapsulated • Highest available level of respiratory, skin, and eye protection from solid, liquid, and gaseous chemicals
B	Worn when the chemical(s) have been identified, but do not require a high level of skin protection	• Liquid-splash protective suit • Offers same level of respiratory protection as Level A but less skin protection • No protection against chemical vapors or gases • Usually worn by decontamination team

C	Used when the type of airborne substance is known and contact with chemical(s) will not affect the skin	• Support function protective garment • Provides same level of skin protection as Level B but a lower level of respiratory protection • Provides liquid-splash protection but no protection against chemical vapors or gases • Not acceptable for use in a chemical emergency response
D	Used when the atmosphere of the involved area contains no known chemical hazards	• Provides no respiratory protection and minimal skin protection • Should not be worn in the hot zone • Not acceptable for use in a chemical emergency response

Hazardous Materials Information Resources

- Your local hazardous materials (Hazmat) response team
- The Chemical Transportation Emergency Center (CHEMTREC) provides a 24-hour hotline: (800) 424-9300. It can provide product and emergency action information.
- The *Emergency Response Guidebook*, published by the U.S. Department of Transportation
- Your regional PCC can provided detailed information, including decontamination methods and treatment.
- Material Safety Data Sheets

Establishing Safety Zones

- Hazardous materials scenes are divided into zones according to safety.

Hot Zone

- The hot zone is the area of the incident that contains the hazardous material (contaminant). This is a dangerous area. The size of the hot zone depends on many factors, including the characteristics of the chemical, the amount released (or spilled or escaped), local weather conditions, the local terrain, and other chemicals in the area.
- Only personnel with high-level PPE enter this area.
- The hot zone is considered contaminated and dangerous until cleared by trained personnel.

Warm Zone

The warm zone is also called the *contamination reduction zone*.

- The warm zone is a controlled area for entry into the hot zone.
- The warm zone is where most operations will take place as a support area for the hot zone. It also serves as the decontamination area for those exiting the hot zone.
- All personnel in the warm zone must wear appropriate protective equipment.

Safe Zone

The safe zone is also called the *cold zone* or *support zone*.

- The safe zone is an area safe from exposure or the threat of exposure.
- This zone serves as the staging area for personnel and equipment.
- If there is no risk to you, remove patients to a safe zone.
- You should not move from this zone or allow anyone else access the scene from this zone unless they have specialized training and PPE.
- The Incident Command Post is located in the cold zone.

START Triage System

- START is an acronym for **S**imple **T**riage **A**nd **R**apid **T**reatment.

- When using the START system, your initial patient assessment and treatment should take less than 30 seconds for each patient.

- Four areas are evaluated during your initial assessment: (1) the ability to walk (ambulation), (2) respirations, (3) perfusion, and (4) mental status.

- On the basis of your assessment findings, you then place the patient into 1 of 4 categories:

  —Red—immediate treatment

  —Yellow—delayed treatment

  —Green—minor (ambulatory patients; "walking wounded")

  —Black—dead or dying

Incident Command System

- The purpose of the National Incident Management System is to provide a consistent nationwide template that allows all governmental, private-sector, and nongovernmental agencies to work together during domestic incidents.

- Examples of domestic incidents include acts of terrorism, wildland and urban fires, floods, hazardous materials spills, nuclear accidents, aircraft accidents, earthquakes, tornadoes, hurricanes, typhoons, and war-related disasters.

- The Incident Command System (ICS) [also called the Incident Management System] is an important part of this comprehensive system.

- ICS is a standardized system developed to assist with the control, direction, and coordination of emergency response resources.

- The ICS can be used at an incident of any type and size, from an everyday call to the large and complex incident.

Advanced Airway Techniques

Endotracheal Intubation: Indications

- Prolonged artificial ventilation is required.
- Adequate artificial ventilation cannot be achieved by other methods.
- The patient is unresponsive and has no cough or gag reflex.
- The patient is unable to protect his own airway (cardiac arrest, unresponsive).
- Respiratory failure has occurred, or there is an impending airway obstruction.

Endotracheal Tube Sizing

- The average size endotracheal (ET) tube for an adult man is 8.0-8.5 mm i.d.
- The average size ET tube for an adult woman is 7-8 mm i.d.
- When selecting the proper size ET tube for the pediatric patient, you should use a length-based tape. The tape provides all recommended ET tube sizes, blade sizes, vital signs, and other information for children who weigh up to about 35 kg.
- If a length-based tape is not available, you can use the following formulas to estimate the correct ET tube size for children 1 to 10 years of age:

  (16 + age in years)/4 or (age in years/4) + 4 = *uncuffed* ET tube size (mm i.d.)

  (age in years/4) + 3 = *cuffed* ET tube size (mm i.d.)

Endotracheal Intubation: Complications

- Slowing of the heart rate. The structures of the upper airway are sensitive to stimulation. Stimulation can cause a slow heart rate, especially in children.
- Soft-tissue trauma to the lips, teeth, tongue, gums, and airway structures
- Inadequate oxygenation because of prolonged or unsuccessful intubation attempts
- Intubation of the right mainstem bronchus
- Intubation of the esophagus
- Removal of the tube by the patient (self-extubation)
- Vomiting and aspiration
- Vocal cord damage
- Obstruction of the tube by secretions
- Swelling of the larynx or trachea

Esophageal-Tracheal Combitube
Indications

- Respiratory arrest
- Cardiac arrest

Contraindications

- Intact gag reflex
- Height less than 4 feet
- Known esophageal disease
- Recent ingestion of a caustic substance
- Known or suspected foreign body obstruction of the larynx or trachea